Herbal
MEDICINE

100 KEY HERBS
WITH ALL THEIR USES AS HERBAL REMEDIES FOR HEALTH AND HEALING

COPYRIGHT 2014 © CHRISTINE ADAMS, M.D.

Disclaimer

The information in this book is not to be used as medical advice. The information presented should be used in combination with guidance from your physician.

All rights reserved. No part of this publication or the information in it may be quoted from or reproduced in any form by means such as printing, scanning, photocopying or otherwise without prior written permission of the copyright holder.

Effort has been made to ensure that the information in this book is accurate and complete, however, the author and the publisher do not warrant the accuracy of the information, text and graphics contained within the book due to the rapidly changing nature of science, research, known and unknown facts and internet. The Author and the publisher do not hold any responsibility for errors, omissions or contrary interpretation of the subject matter herein. This book is presented solely for motivational and informational purposes only.

Table of Contents

Introduction 4

Chapter 1: Herbal Medicine Preparation ... 10

Chapter 2: Classes of Herbal Medicines 13

Chapter 3: How to Store and Take Herbal Medicines 19

Chapter 4: Common Medicinal Herbs and Their Uses 22

Chapter 5: Flower Remedies 88

Conclusion 95

Introduction

The medicinal use of herbs and other parts of plants predates Western medicine and most of the other healing traditions, such as Chinese and Indian medicine. Medicinal plants were and are frequently used to treat both acute and chronic conditions in Traditional Chinese and Ayurvedic medicine, and surprisingly similar plant remedies have been used by native North and South American practitioners. Herbal medicine entered Western medical history around the time of Hippocrates, and herbs were used from the 5th century BCE on, not only to alleviate the manifestations of a particular disease but to balance the basic types of body fluids or humors and to strengthen the body's inherent resistance to disease and stimulate its restorative capacity once illness started.

Greek physicians first used many of the medicinal plants available to them, such as fennel, rosemary and saffron, and Greek practitioners were commissioned by Alexander the Great and several Roman emperors to travel with their respective armies to study potentially useful healing practices and bring back potentially useful plant remedies from other lands. Theophrastus, who published *An Enquiry on Plants* under the auspices of Alexander, and Dioscorides, who wrote the first *Materia Medica* at the time of Nero, described hundreds of medicinal plants, many of which are still in use today. Many of the ancient herbalist's discoveries survived the fall of Rome and became widely used in the Middle Ages, such as basil, garlic, parsley and peppermint; the *Leech Book of Bald* from the reign of Alfred the Great in England, for example, described several hundred plants used to treat disease. Other knowledge was preserved by Arab physicians during Europe's dark ages, and advances such as the chemical equipment used to prepare herbal and other medicines and methods for distilling plant essences and diffusing them in the air, can be traced to Rhazes, Avicenna and other Islamic scholars.

During the medieval period, doctors began to concoct combinations of plant, mineral and even animal material that sought to treat disease more aggressively, often by inducing purging or vomiting and sometimes doing more harm than good. These prescriptions, as they came to be called, became the prerogative of trained doctors, licensed first by the universities and guilds of physicians and surgeons and then by government authorities. Self-care by interested and knowledgeable individuals and the use of traditional and usually herbal medicines was at first discouraged and later condemned; it has been suggested that one of the driving forces behind the periodic witch hunts in most European countries between the 13th and 17th century was the desire of the medical establishments of the day to remove from influence those people, often women, who had knowledge of healing and herbs. A more enlightened attitude was eventually grudgingly adopted by orthodox physicians, perhaps beginning in the 15th century with the Swiss doctor and alchemist Theophrastus Bombastus von Hohenheim, who called himself

Paracelsus. Paracelsus and his adherents advocated the use of gentler and less toxic remedies for disease, often of herbal origin, and suggested that plants and the medicines derived from them contained life force or energy that could be transferred to the sick with beneficial effect. Paracelsus was not always right in his theories: he enunciated the "doctrine of signatures", which stated that God gave man clues as to the medicinal use of plants through their shape and appearance, which is not always true, but he and his school did in a way begin to reunite Western and Eastern approaches to healing. He did not always see it that way, and in fact burned the old-fashioned works of Galen and Avicenna during colorful and combative public lectures on modern medicine. Paracelsus was also the originator of the idea that, rather than alchemists trying to turn "base substances" into gold, "chemists" should try to identify the active principles in curative plants and purify them for use as medicine; this gave rise to the discipline that is today called pharmacology, and to the continuing search for synthetic chemical drugs.

Herbal medicine established a strong presence in the English-speaking countries, and the first *Herball, or General Historie of Plantes* was published in London in 1597 by John Gerard. Nicholas Culpeper's *The English Physician* from 1652 is still read today, although it attempts in places to combine plant medicines with astrology and the zodiac. European physicians became more interested in drugs, the word coming from the Dutch *drogge* (to grind up), but herbal healing was transferred to the New Word, where it met an active tradition of native healing with plants and became part of the natural or eclectic method taught during the 19th century at many

American medical schools. The development of chemistry in the 19th century, particularly in Germany, led to the growth of a pharmaceutical industry closely tied to the medical profession and to "scientific" medical practice and education, and to the rapid development of many safe and highly effective chemical medicines, and some that were not; during 1897, for example, the same team at Bayer in Barmen, Germany synthesized, tested and introduced arguably the most successful drug in history (aspirin), an important if sometimes problematic drug (paracetamol or acetaminophen, known as Tylenol) and perhaps the most disastrous drug of all time (heroin). Herbal and other natural medicines came to be suspected and even derided as less consistent, less effective and less safe.

The growth of medical science and education at European universities led the Rockefeller interests and the Carnegie Foundation to commission Abraham Flexner in 1907 to study American medical schools and recommend means of improving them. Although Flexner was not a physician, had not finished graduate studies at Harvard and the University of Berlin, and had in fact never been inside a medical school, he produced in 1910 a highly influential report that ushered in the modern era of medical education and practice, oriented toward surgery and synthetic drugs, conducted at large hospitals and universities, closely allied with the pharmaceutical industry and heavily regulated by the State. The homeopathic, naturopathic and eclectic medical schools closed, the herbalists retreated to farms and forests and only a handful of "alternative" doctors, for example 75 homeopathic physicians, were in practice in the United States by the middle of the 20th century. More importantly, Western and particularly American medicine became increasingly focused on "health" as the absence of diagnosable disease and "health care" as the eradication of symptoms as they arose.

About 80 per cent of the world's population has continued to rely largely and sometimes entirely on natural sources of medicines, particularly plants, and healing systems other than conventional Western medicine have continued to operate in eastern countries and areas like South America and Africa where resources for health care are more limited. European physicians did not turn so completely from natural or herbal treatments as did their American counterparts, and alternative, complementary or holistic medical techniques are offered by as many as one-third of practitioners. A variety of factors in the United States have contributed to the resurgence during the second half of the 20th century of consumer-oriented and often patient-directed health care with a greater emphasis on health maintenance and the importance of balance and well-being. The rise of the New Age movement, increasing skepticism of experts and authorities in light of recent history and the relationship between alternative life styles and alternative pharmaceuticals have been suggested, as has the rapid increase in cost occasioned by the rapid acceleration of scientific medicine and the recognition after about a century that synthetic drugs are not always a panacea and conventional medicine is not always effective. It is likely that a balance between modern science and traditional healing methods is now reasserting itself, and this will be beneficial for the management of chronic illnesses.

9

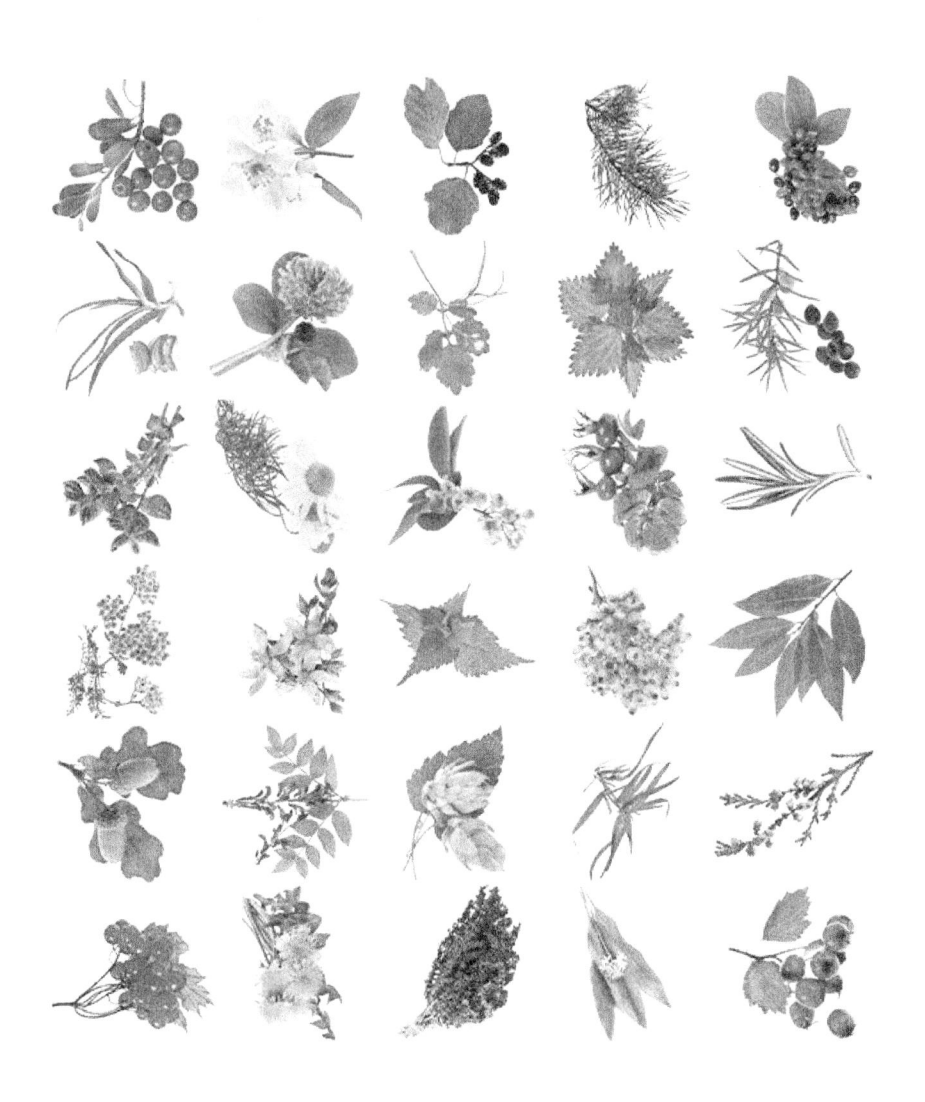

Chapter 1
HERBAL MEDICINE PREPARATION

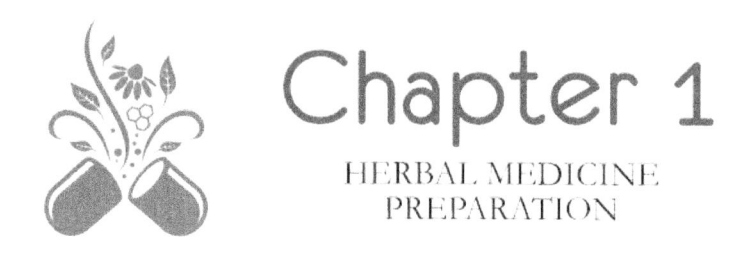

"Herbs" are the aerial parts of plants, that is, the portions of the plant that can be seen above the ground. This includes the flowers, stem and leaves; the roots are not classed as herbs, although herbalists and natural medicine practitioners often make use of roots in therapeutic preparations. There are several ways to take herbs orally. The chopped or ground herbal parts of the plant are most commonly preserved in water and alcohol, which is a *tincture*. Homeopathic medicines begin as a "mother tincture" which is then repeatedly diluted, and other tinctures are easily assimilated. Alcohol is sometimes used to extract constituents from plants, but for those who do not like the taste of an alcohol-based tincture or do not wish to take alcohol, the alcohol can be removed by dilution and evaporation with hot water and the remaining mixture can be added to juice or glycerin. Dried herb powder can be placed in a *capsule* and swallowed, often the most convenient preparation, or the capsule can be opened and the powder placed in food, water or juice. *Tablets* are made by compressing the powdered material, which makes it more compact but not always congenial to swallow.

A dissolvable **lozenge** will sometimes address this problem. A cloth can also be saturated with powdered or dissolved herb, and applied hot, warm or cold to the skin as a *compress. Tea* is for many people the most convenient way of giving or taking herbal medicines, and may be made as either a *decoction* or an *infusion.* An infusion, made by immersing the herb in hot water, uses the softer parts of herbs like leaves and flowers, either as powder or in a tea bag, usually sitting for 10 to 15 minutes in a cup of boiling water. A decoction, used for harder parts like bark, roots and seeds, involves placing the herb in boiling water, simmering for 15 to 25 minutes and then steeping for 10 or so minutes. If a tea bag is not available, 1 tablespoon of dried herb or 3 tablespoons of fresh herb are usually used for a cup of water.

Herbs can be applied to the skin, especially when inflamed, through a cloth soaked in an infusion or decoction (*fomentation*). The *essential oils* of many plants can be extracted with water or distilled with steam, then applied to the skin, diluted with sweet almond, jojoba or some other oil so as not to cause irritation. The volatile oils can also be evaporated and inhaled. An emulsion of water and oil can be used to make an herb *cream* and applied topically, the herb extract or herb oil can be combined with beeswax to make a *salve* or the powdered herb can be suspended in oil as a *liniment*. If plant material is ground and made into a paste, then placed between two thin pieces of cloth an applied to the skin, this is a *poultice.* Herb oils can be added to *steaming* hot water, particularly for chest and respiratory problems, or can be dissolved in a *bath* (usually the essential oil) for general skin application at a low dose or given rectally as a *suppository* for entry into the bloodstream.

Plant medicines are sometimes harder to standardize than laboratory-synthesized chemicals, and this was one reason pharmaceutical drugs came to be preferred over herbal preparations. It is often possible to get a plant extract standardized to contain a specific amount of the active ingredient that has the desired therapeutic effect, and this is preferable whenever possible. This cannot always be done, however, as the active constituent or constituents of a particular herb are not always known despite long clinical experience with the plant.

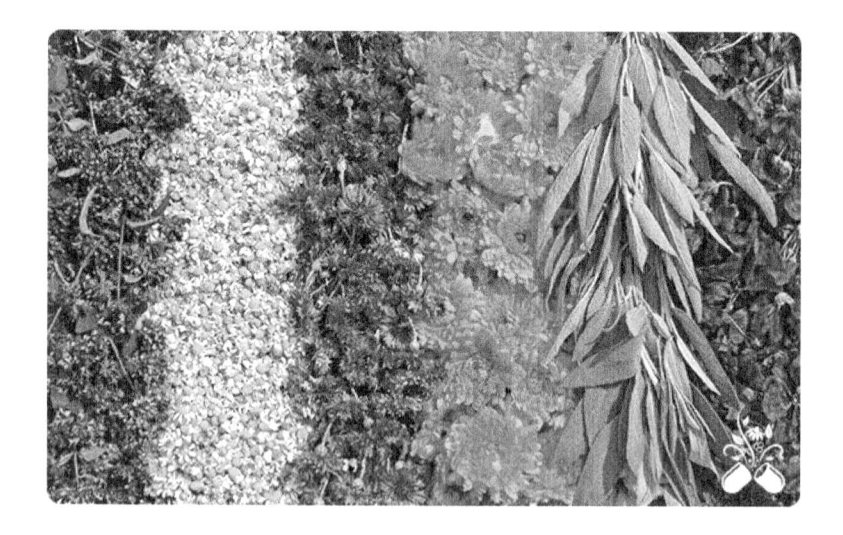

Chapter 2
CLASSES OF HERBAL MEDICINES

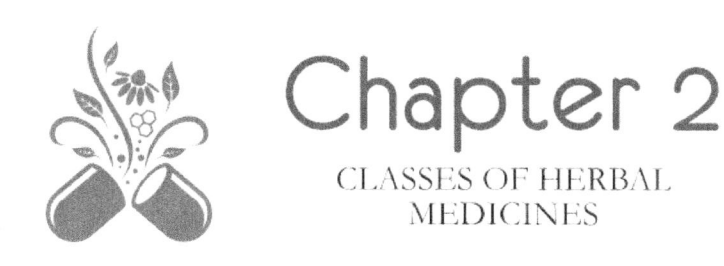

Thousands of kinds of leaves, berries, flowers, stems and roots have been used as medicines over the centuries, too many to summarize in even cursory detail. Herbal medicines for diabetes and metabolic syndrome will be considered shortly. There are numerous classes of herbal medicines, chiefly based on their properties and actions. In more or less alphabetical order, some of the important ones are as follows.

Abortifacients are plants that cause miscarriages, and must of course be avoided in pregnant women or those contemplating it; pennyroyal is an example.

Adaptogens help the body adapt to stress and support or restore normal levels of life force or energy; such a plant is often called a "tonic", and often work by enhancing adrenal gland function, exemplified by ginseng.

An *alterative* improves general health, often through enhancing the digestion and absorption of nutrients or facilitating the breakdown and excretion of toxins; such plants are sometimes called "blood purifiers", and burdock root is an example.

Anodyne or analgesic herbs relieve pain; an example is white willow, from which the active ingredient of aspirin was first isolated. Herbs like goldenseal that decrease the production of nasal and respiratory tract mucus, congestion with which used to be called "catarrh", are termed *anticatarrhals*.

Antidepressants are herbs that lift depression, such as St. John's wort, and usually enhance levels of serotonin and norepinephrine in the brain.

An *antidote* counteracts the effects of a plant or animal poison, and an *antiemetic* counteracts the urge to vomit, either from stomach or intestinal disorder or untoward stimulation of vomiting centers in the brain stem.

***Antifungal* herbs** prevent the establishment of fungal infections or kill fungi when infection is present. Herbs that reduce or stop the inappropriate production of breast milk (galactorrhea), which can be a symptom of breast disease, hormonal imbalance, drug effect or pituitary gland tumor, are referred to as *antigalactics* (e.g., sage). Black walnut, garlic and wormwood are examples of *antihelminthics* or *antiparasitics*, which destroy worms and parasites.

***Anti-inflammatory* herbs** antagonize the various chemical transmitters that initiate or maintain inflammation in the body, and are exemplified by black cohosh, boswellia, bromelain and licorice root.

***Antimicrobial* herbs** kill or disrupt the growth of bacteria. *Antioxidants* protect cells from oxidation, chemical reactions in which cells are damaged by toxic atoms with extra electrons (free radicals); there are many of these in common use, chiefly astragalus, ginkgo, hawthorn berry, milk thistle, thyme and wild oregano. *Antipyretic* herbs such as yarrow reduce fever. Antiseptic herbs like calendula or propolis prevent growth of bacteria on the skin. Black cohosh, chamomile, kava, valerian and wild yam are examples of *antispasmodic* herbs that alleviate muscle spasms. Many over-the-counter cough drops contain *antitussive* herbs, chiefly horehound and wild cherry bark. Tumor growth is suppressed or stopped by *antitumor* herbs such as astragalus and echinacea.

Astringents constrict or contract tissue, and may therefore stop bleeding or diarrhea; examples include geranium, witch hazel, sage and yarrow.

Bitters taste bitter and stimulate the digestive tract, and thereby increase appetite when low but apparently do not foster overeating; they also enhance digestion and absorption, and burdock root, dandelion root, gentian root and goldenseal are examples. *Bronchodilator* herbs dilate and relax the bronchial tree in the lungs, and are for that reason useful in asthma, bronchitis, cough and chronic lung disease. Examples include peppermint and yerba santa.

Calmative herbs are gently calming and relaxing, and include chamomile, hops, kava, passionflower and valerian. The *carminative* herbs, such as anise, fennel, ginger and peppermint) reduce or prevent gas. An herb that stimulates bowel evacuation is a *cathartic* laxative (e.g., cascara sagrada, rhubarb or senna). *Cholagogue* herbs stimulate bile release from the gallbladder, exemplified by dandelion root, while *choleretic* herbs like burdock, dandelion and milk thistle cause increased bile production by the liver.

Demulcent **herbs** heal and lubricate irritated mucous membranes, and are exemplified by slippery elm. A *diaphoretic* herb, such as boneset or yarrow, causes perspiration and is helpful for colds and viral infections. Dandelion and parsley are examples of *diuretic* herbs, which promote urination.

Emetic **herbs** induce vomiting, and some like ipecac are still in common use. *Expectorants* promote the expulsion of mucus from the respiratory tract; examples include horehound, lungwort and yerba santa. White willow, also a pain reliever, is an example of a *febrifuge*, an herb that reduces fever.

Herbs that stimulate rather than reduce the flow of breast milk, helpful in difficult nursing, are *galactagogues* (e.g., blessed thistle, fennel and fenugreek).

A *hemostatic* **herb** like cinnamon or yarrow helps to stop bleeding. *Hepatic* herbs stimulate the liver to increase metabolism and produce bile; some of these are the choleretic herbs mentioned above, but the class also includes artichoke, licorice and yellow dock. Valerian is a widely-used example of *hypnotic* herbs, that induce generally natural sleep. A number of herbs are effective for high blood pressure, such as garlic and hawthorn berry, and these are classed as *hypotensive.*

Laxatives are the most widely used family of herbs today, and include the cathartics like senna and also those that encourage fecal expulsion more gently by relaxation or lubrication, such as aloe and rehmania. A *lymphagogue* stimulates flow in the lymph ducts and filtering by the lymph glands, which assists clearing of toxins; examples are burdock, ceanothus and pokeroot.

***Mucolytic* herbs** thin mucus secretions, and are essentially the same as the anticatarrhal herbs mentioned above.

A relaxing and elevating herb such as chamomile, lavender, passionflower, skullcap and valerian can also be categorized as a *nervine*, and these have historically been used to treat anxiety. Some herbs have excellent nutritional value and can be used as dietary supplements; nettle is an example of such a *nutritive*.

***Palliative* treatment** in conventional medicine alleviates symptoms but does not cure the underlying disease; this term was first used to describe herbal treatments like white willow for pain or passionflower for sleep. Some herbs also have *prophylactic* uses in preventing disease, such as bitter melon and possibly gingko for circulatory problems.

***Rubefacient* herbs** irritate the skin and mucous membranes, and increase blood flow and drain congestion; an example is the well-known effect of horseradish on the sinuses.

***Sedative* herbs** calm during the day and facilitate sleep at night, and the term is interchangeable with nervine, calmative and hypnotic. *Stimulant* herbs have an awakening and enlivening effect, exemplified by the several kinds of ginseng used in Western herbalism and Chinese medicine, as well as ashwagandha in the Indian tradition. A *synergist* herb increases the effectiveness of another herb, so that the combined effect of both is greater than the sum of the two actions; licorice root is an example of this.

Many herbs are *tonics*, in that they enhance function generally (e.g. ginseng) or strengthen or normalize the function of a particular organ or system (e.g. milk thistle for the liver and pokeroot for the lymphatic system).

A **vermifuge** aids in the expulsion of worms, and is thus the same as an antihelminthic; wormwood derived its name from this action. *Vulnerary* herbs promote tissue healing, such as aloe for burns and irritation, arnica for bruises and contusions and calendula for cuts and scrapes.

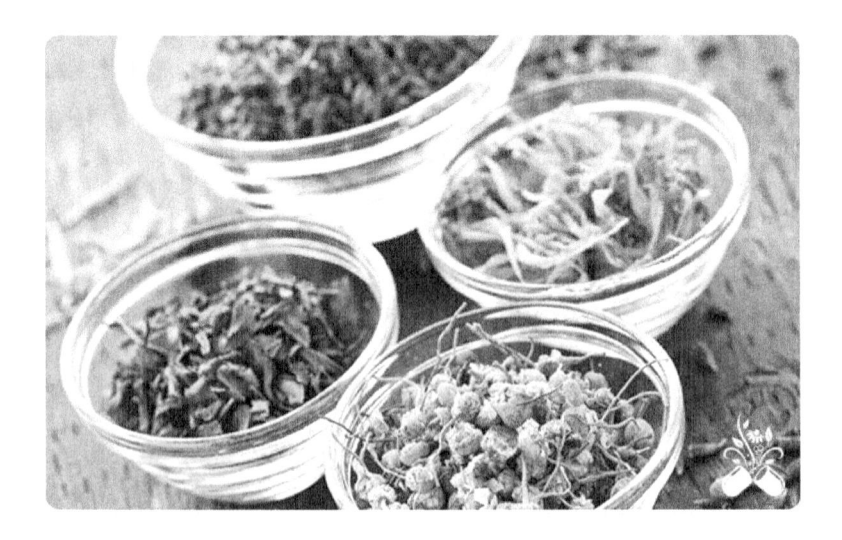

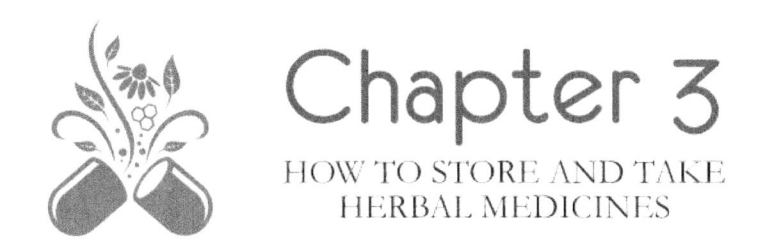

Chapter 3
HOW TO STORE AND TAKE HERBAL MEDICINES

Herbal preparations are in general quite safe, although some plants with medicinal uses are toxic and others actually poisonous. These cannot be sold to the public but may be found in the wild; it is therefore important to know the identity of a plant with certainty before harvesting and using it. It is also advisable to know the area from which the plants are obtained, and to be familiar with the people who gather them, in order to feel confident that safe plants are being distinguished from unsafe ones. It may be helpful to seek the advice of an herbalist before using wild plants, and some herbalists oppose the use of wild plants for medical purposes because many medicinal species are or are becoming endangered. Some of the toxic and poisonous plants may safely be taken in homeopathic preparations as described above. Commercially purchased herbs should indicate dosages and give directions, and ingredients should be listed in order of potency. The specific part of the plant that has been used should also be listed; in some plants the leaves have medicinal properties but not the roots or stem while in others the stem may be effective but not the leaves or roots, and still others have their active ingredients in the root. Herbs should be fresh and indicate an expiration date, and should be wrapped and sealed; ideally, the lot number should also be listed, in case some contaminant or other problem is later identified. Organic herbs are preferable, so that the effects of herbicides and pesticides should be avoided.

Commercial herbs are easier to store than those obtained in the wild. Bulk herbs should be kept in airtight glass containers, out of direct light and at a constant temperature of 55 to 65° F (12-18°C). Tinctures should be stored in upright bottles in a cupboard, out of the light. Tablets and capsules should be in closed containers and not in hot or humid places. Loose teas and tea bags should be kept dry, out of the light, and with as little air exposure as possible.

Herbs, like almost everything else, should be stored out of the reach of children. Children can be safely treated with herbs, however, but may need some help getting them down on account of the taste or texture and usually require smaller doses than adults. The alcohol used to make many tinctures may be evaporated by mixing the desired herb in ¼ cup of hot water for 5 minutes, and when cool the tinctured water can be mixed with juice or water; this approach also works for herbal teas. The contents of capsules can be mixed with preferred foods, a 50-50 mixture of tincture and water can be dropped into juice or the desired amount of herbal preparation can be squirted into the mouth with a dropper. One common recommendation for dosing is to give 20 per cent of the adult dose to a 5-30 pound (2.3-13.6 kg) child, 25 per cent for 30-60 pounds (13.6-27.2 kg), one-third of the dose if the child weights 60 to 90 pounds (27.2-40.8 kg), half of the adult dose for 90 to 120 pounds (40.8-54.4 kg) and 75 per cent if 120-150 pounds (54.4-68.3 kg).

There is some difference of opinion about when and how often to take herbal medicines. For an acute problem, a dose every 2 to 3 waking hours is recommended, in order to support the body's ongoing response to an illness. The herbal preparation should be continued for 2 days after resolution of symptoms, particularly for an infection. Chronic conditions are best managed with 2-3 times a day dosing. Herbs that strengthen digestion, such as bitters should be taken before meals, and taking herbs with meals may be helpful if the herbs upset the stomach; otherwise the herbs may be better absorbed if taken between meals.

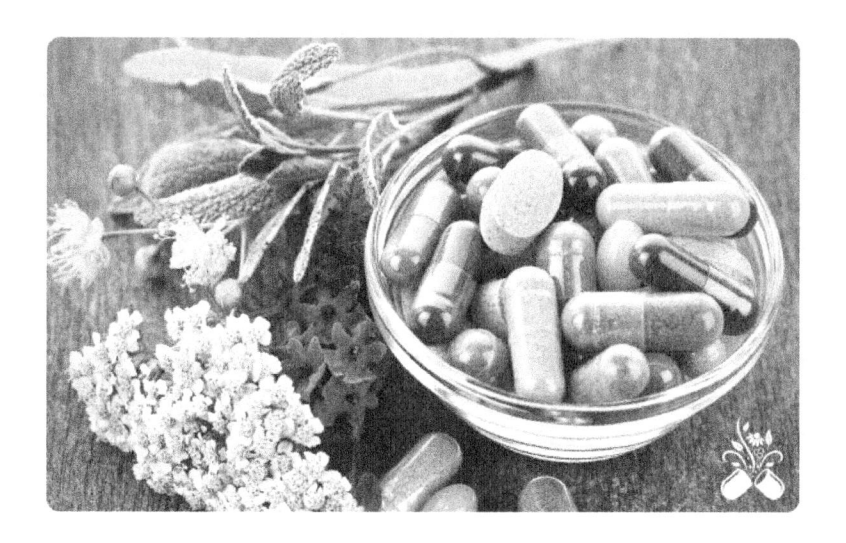

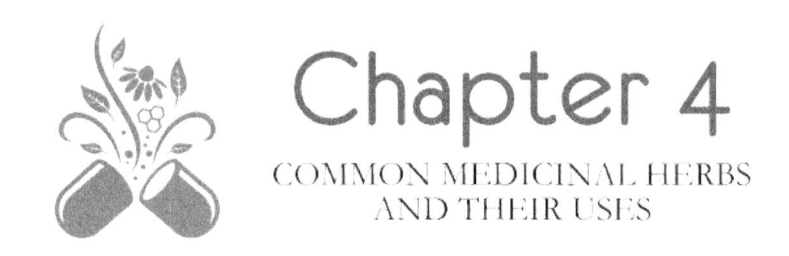

Chapter 4
COMMON MEDICINAL HERBS AND THEIR USES

Alfalfa *(Medicago sativa)* is commonly used for detoxification, balancing of hormonal effects and to alkalinize blood and urine. The leaves and less frequently the seeds are used, either in bulk or ground and put in capsules or tablets. Alfalfa is highly nutritious and can be eaten, although it is not too often used as food. It is effective for anemia, arthritis, asthma high cholesterol, diabetes, indigestion, menstrual disturbances and menopausal symptoms, peptic ulcer disease, skin disorders and various urinary tract disorders, particularly infections, bladder stones and prostatitis. It appears to lower cholesterol by preventing cholesterol absorption in the gut, and can increase the activity of the immune system, so can worsen or possibly precipitate symptoms of autoimmune disorders such as multiple sclerosis, systemic lupus erythematosus and rheumatoid arthritis. Alfalfa can also have an estrogen-like effect, and is for this reason inadvisable for pregnant women and a potential problem for some hormone-sensitive conditions like fibroids, endometriosis and cancers of the breast, uterus or ovaries. Photosensitivity has occasionally been reported, so sunblock is appropriate to use when outside.

Aloe *(Aloe vera)* is one of the most potent healing herbs for the skin and digestive tract, and can be taken internally as juice or applied topically. It is commonly used externally for burns, scrapes, canker sores and skin irritation, and has been effective internally for *Candida* infections, constipation, inflammatory bowel disease, intestinal infections, ulcers and a variety of other digestive disorders. It has also helped topically with psoriasis and the intestinal complications of diabetes and HIV infection. The leaves are customarily used, either as a source of juice for internal use or macerated or ground to make gels, creams and salves; the juice is often used in topical preparations, and it is important to use food-grade juice internally. Aloe vera latex, fluid derived from the inner lining of the leaves, was first used as a laxative but can no longer be sold for this purpose; the latex is occasionally used to lower blood sugar levels in diabetes, but its use is discouraged because it can cause hepatitis and hypothyroidism and is unsafe in pregnancy.

Anise *(Pimpinella anisum)* has a sweet taste and is often used to blend with otherwise unpalatable herbs. The seeds are used in cooking, and to make tinctures and teas that have long been prescribed in eastern and western herbalism for bronchitis, cough, colic, digestive disorders of many kinds and parasitic infections. It has no significant adverse effects.

Artichoke *(Cynara scolymus)* is widely eaten, and the leaves are also ground and compounded in capsules or made into tinctures for liver disorders, high cholesterol and fat malabsorption due to diseases of the pancreas, gallbladder or bile duct. Artichokes have among the highest antioxidant contents of vegetables, and increase "good" HDL cholesterol while lowering the "bad" LDL. They also contain the beneficial plant phenols apigenin and luteolin, and serve as a probiotic by promoting the growth of the useful species of *bifidobacteria*. Cyanarine from the pulp of the leaves is an effective non-sugar sweetener, and is sometimes used as a less bitter "bitter" for digestive problems, as well as an ingredient in cocktails, particularly in Europe. There are no major adverse effects reported, but large amounts at once may cause loose stools, and because it is a cholagogue and increases bile flow; people with bile duct obstruction best avoid it.

Ashwagandha *(Withania somniferum)* is an Indian member of the nightshade family and a relative of tomatoes and potatoes; it has long been used in Ayurvedic medicine, and is recognized in western herbalism as a blood, nervous system and immune tonic. The roots and leaves contain steroid-like lactone compounds, but the roots are primarily used, ground and prepared as tinctures or put in capsules. It is highly effective for stress and anxiety, and has been shown more effective than psychotherapy in some controlled trials, with few or no adverse effects. It can also reduce fatigue, increase energy and enhance exercise tolerance, and has been reported to be effective for the physiological consequences of aging, anemia, chronic fatigue syndrome, immune system compromise, memory disorders and osteoarthritis.

Astralagus *(Astralagus membranaceus or A. propinquus)* is an Asian perennial plant that is one of the 50 fundamental herbs of traditional Chinese medicine. It is known in China as *huang qi, bei qi* or *huang hua huang qi,* and is a general tonic particularly useful for diabetes. It improves lung, adrenal gland and gastrointestinal functioning, promotes sweating, enhances glucose metabolism, facilitates wound healing and reduces fatigue. An extract of the plant increases telomerase, an enzyme involved in DNA repair, and this may prevent cell death and have a variety of beneficial effects. The roots contain saponins and isoflavones, and it is therefore an adaptogen with general benefit when under stress as well as an enhancer of immune function. The roots are used in tinctures or teas and are compounded in capsules, and the herb is recommended for immune support and general health as well as diarrhea, diabetes fatigue, heart disease, hepatitis, hypertension, kidney disease and prevention of the consequences of cancer chemotherapy and radiation treatment. Because of its immune effects, it has been used in HIV infection to prevent the emergence of AIDS, and it may protect against the common cold and other viral infections. It has sometimes been used to increase blood flow to the skin and foster wound healing. It is best to avoid *Astralagus* with a fever because of its effects on skin blood flow and sweating, but it has been suggested to help certain cancers (breast, cervical and lung) in combination with glossy privet (*Ligustrum lucidum*). There are several other members of the *Astralagus* family that contain a toxic alkaloid (swainsonine) that has been linked to animal poisonings; these species are not usually present in preparations used by humans, but it is best to make certain that a preparation contains only the *membranaceus* type.

Barberry *(Berberis vulgaris)* is a widespread shrub with very tart berries that are eaten or made into jam in Europe. The plant is mildly poisonous except for its fruits and seeds, and cannot be grown in or imported into the

United States because it is a host species for the wheat rust fungus that is a serious threat to food grains. The dried roots and bark may be imported, however, and are prepared as tinctures or put into capsules, and can be made into an ointment for topical use. It is soothing to the skin and stimulates the immune system, so has been used for general immune support and to treat *Candida* and parasitic infections as well as diarrhea, eczema and psoriasis. It should not be given to infants or used in pregnancy or when breastfeeding because of its mild toxicity.

Basil *(Ocimum basilicum)* was formerly called St. Joseph's wort, and although native to India, has been cultivated in the West for thousands of years and is one of the most commonly-used cooking spices. In many cultures, it has been put in the hands or mouths of the dead to ensure a safe passage to the afterlife. It was used medicinally by the ancient Greeks and is a potent antioxidant as well as an antibacterial and antiviral agent. Its seeds and leaves are used to make tinctures, tablets and capsules, and it has been given for asthma, diabetes and stress in India, and for constipation, diabetes, various digestive disorders and hypothyroidism in the West. It can decrease platelet aggregation and clot formation as well as tumor growth in mice, and so may prove to be useful for the treatment of vascular disease and cancer. These potential effects warrant caution during pregnancy and breastfeeding, and it is also recommended to avoid Basil with liver and kidney disease.

Bilberry *(Vaccinium myrtillus)* is a European relative of the blueberry, widely used in jam. British authorities during World War II observed that some Royal Air Force crews had remarkably good accuracy in bombing raids over Germany, and found that these crews tended to eat bilberry jam at breakfast. This led to more systematic studies in England that found the herb to be highly beneficial for eye health, although the U.S. Navy has not been able to confirm this recently. Nevertheless, the berries as tea, tincture, capsules or tablets have been used with benefit for cataracts, eyestrain, glaucoma, macular degeneration, poor night vision, and retinopathy, as well as other complications of diabetes, diarrhea, hemorrhoids and varicose veins. There are no reported adverse effects.

Bitter melon *(Momordica charantia)* is a tropical and subtropical member of the gourd family that is bitter in taste and has some toxic parts such as seed coverings, that can even cause fatal poisoning in children. The leaves and shoots are safe as greens, however, and the fruit is safe when cooked and is widely used as a bitter flavor in Asian and Caribbean cooking and sometimes put in Chinese beer in place of hops. The fruit is also used in Asian and African medicine, and tinctures, capsules or tablets are particularly effective for diabetes. Bitter melon enhances insulin production and effect, and may reduce diabetic complications; there is also some evidence that the fruit may impede the progression of cancer. Excessive doses can result in abdominal pain and diarrhea.

Black cohosh *(Cimcifuga* or *Acataea racemosa)* is part of the exceeding numerous family of *Ranunculaceae,* which includes clematis, wolfbane, goldenseal and passionflower and grows almost everywhere in North America. Black cohosh is sometimes called "bugbane" because its flowers have a mildly medicinal smell that repels insects. Many plants in this family are poisonous, such as wolfbane or aconite, but have long been used medicinally by native Americans, and in high dilution are also effective homeopathic remedies. Black cohosh roots and rhizomes have been used since Precolumbian times in the New World for various gynecologic symptoms, particularly menopause and menstrual cramps, pain and irritability. The roots and rhizomes (underground stems) are used for capsules and tablets, or are ground to make tinctures. Arthritis, depression and fibromyalgia and other types of chronic pain have also been treated with benefit. The plant contains estrogen-like compounds which are probably responsible for its effects on menopause and menstrual problems, but several compounds that bind to serotonin receptors and may be analogues of this important neurotransmitter have also been found, which suggest more widespread effect. Triterpene glycosides are also present, and these compounds may protect against bone breakdown and the development of osteoporosis. Because of its hormonal effects, it should not be used when pregnant or breastfeeding.

Bladderwrack *(Fusus vesiculosus)* is a seaweed sometimes called "black tang" or "rockweed", and grows widely in both Atlantic and Pacific waters. This was found to contain iodine in 1811, and became the first widely-used treatment for goiter. It is still one of the most common herbal treatments for thyroid disease, and is also used for digestive upset, particularly constipation. This is a source of many minerals in addition to iodine, but can also contain many toxins and contaminants so a carefully-screened and well-cleaned product is needed. The stem is used to make tea or tincture, or is dried and ground for capsules and tablets. There are no reported adverse effects if toxins and contaminants are avoided.

Black walnut *(Juglans nigra)* is a flowering tree native to the eastern United States, and secretes a toxic substance (juglone) into the soil that inhibits the respiration of other plants and retards their competition. The nuts can be toxic to horses and humans, but the dried husks are used to make tinctures and capsules that can safely be taken for short periods in low doses. Black walnut can prevent or treat yeast or parasitic infections, but the American Cancer Society does not accept its reported use in cancer treatment. Large doses over time are a circulatory depressant, and it should not be taken during pregnancy. It is best to have the guidance of a naturopathic physician or medical herbalist when using Black Walnut.

Blessed thistle *(Cnicus benedictus)* is the leaves, stems and flowers of a Mediterranean thistle considered to be a weed in North America, and is a galactogogue which promotes the secretion of breast milk. It is widely used to help nursing mothers, and is also part of several bitters formulas that are used for digestive problems such as constipation and indigestion. In addition to such bitters, it can be steeped in a tea or made into capsules, and has no known adverse effects but as it stimulates lactation it should be avoided during pregnancy.

Blue cohosh *(Caulophyllum thalictroides)* is from a different genus than the black variety, but has also been used by native Americans and later by European midwives for menstrual problems and also as an abortive and contraceptive. The roots and flowers are ground to prepare a tincture or packed in capsules, and are best used for hormonal problems under the guidance of an herbal practitioner, particularly during pregnancy. Headache, high blood pressure and nausea are common side effects, and usually lessen if the dose is decreased.

Boswellia *(Boswellia serrata)* is a genus of trees with fragrant resin, that has been used since ancient times for medicinal purposes, particularly as an anti-inflammatory. The Biblical frankincense was most likely an extract of the tree *Boswellia sacra*, and the resin is today made into capsules and tablets with few or no adverse effects. The major components of the resin, boswellic acids, inhibit the production of leukotrienes, mediators of inflammation that were first discovered in white blood cells (leukocytes) but are present in most other types of cell, and as such prevent the initiation of the inflammatory response that is involved in all sorts of diseases. They also activate apoptosis, or programmed cell death, which is a normal part of the cell life cycle that fails to occur in certain kinds of cancers, resulting in excessive and disorderly proliferation of cells; this may make boswellic acids effective against the growth of cancers, and there is some evidence that they can have a protective effect on liver cells and retard the inflammation that initiates asthma attacks. Boswellia is now widely used for arthritis, asthma, injury and inflammation and ulcerative colitis.

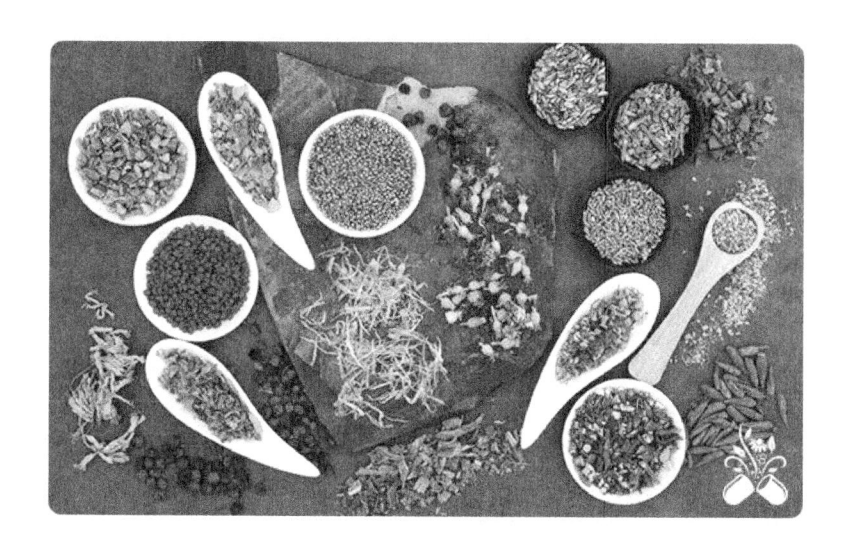

Bromelain is another potent natural anti-inflammatory which is usually derived from the stems of pineapples but which consists chiefly of protein-digesting enzymes (proteases) that are present in all parts of the plant and its fruit. The name is derived from the family to which pineapples belong (*Bromeliaceae*) and the extract was first identified in 1891 and purified in 1892; it has been used as a therapeutic supplement since 1957, and is considered by the National Institutes of Health to be effective for osteoarthritis when taken together with the enzymes trypsin and rutin, a combination which is marked as Phlogenzym. It is felt possibly effective for post-exercise muscle soreness, but is widely used in most other countries as well as in the United States for burns, systemic symptoms of cancer, cardiovascular disease, inadequate protein digestion, prostatitis, recovery from surgery, respiratory infections producing excessive mucus, thrombophlebitis and varicose veins. It is best taken as tablets or capsules between meals to improve absorption, and should not be combined with anticoagulants because it has mild blood-thinning effects.

Bugleweed *(Lycopus virginicus)* or gypsywort is a widely distributed American and European genus of perennial flowering plants that grow along streams and in wetlands. The name "gypsy" comes from the black dye prepared from the juice of *Lycopus europaeus*, which the Roma or gypsies used to darken their skin. The plant was used by medieval apothecaries as an astringent, a cardiac tonic and a nervous system sedative. The leaves and flowers are currently used to make tinctures and capsules for the treatment of hyperthyroidism, and it is sometimes used for anxiety, contraception, heart palpitations and tuberculosis. It should be avoided if pregnant or nursing, and by those with hypothyroidism.

Burdock *(Arctium lappa)* is a European member of the aster/daisy/sunflower family *(Asteraceae)* that has prickly seed-disbursing burrs that catch on fur and clothing and by doing so inspired the Swiss engineer Georges de Mestral to invent Velcro in 1948. The burrs can cause hairballs in cats and can be fatal to birds, who cannot disentangle their feathers. The green portions above ground can cause contact dermatitis in humans, but the roots can be eaten as a vegetable, particularly in Chinese, Japanese or Korean cuisine. The English drank burdock and dandelion mead in ancient times, and it is still a widely consumed soft drink today. Burdock is usually prepared as tincture or capsules for general detoxification. It is particularly good for skin conditions such as acne and rashes, enhances liver function and is an antimicrobial. It contains healthful phystosterols and long-chain essential fatty acids, and is used in Europe for skin and scalp problems, while in traditional Chinese medicine it is called *niubangzhi* and used as a diuretic, diaphoretic and blood purifier.

Butcher's Broom *(Ruscus aculeatus)* is an evergreen shrub that is often seen in gardens, and has long been used for vascular problems. The roots and stems are ground for tablets and capsules or suspended in a tincture, and cause few adverse effects, chiefly occasional nausea. There is considerable evidence that the plant is medically useful. It increases blood flow to brain and limbs, so has been used for cerebrovascular insufficiency and cardiovascular disease. It strengthens capillary walls and has been found effective for varicose veins. Commission E of the German BAM, an agency which is equivalent to the American FDA, approves and regulates the sale of herbal and other natural health products and has approved Butcher's Broom for the treatment of hemorrhoids.

Calendula, the marigold, is formally called *Calendula "officinalis"* because it has been in so many formularies of approved medicinal plants over the centuries. The name "calendula" derives from the Latin for "little clock", apparently because of its appearance, and "marigold" refers to the Virgin Mary, because the flowers were so often used to decorate Her statues. The flowers are similarly used to decorate the images of Hindu deities, and *Calendula* has long been used in both eastern and western cooking and herbal medicine. The flowers have often been used on the battlefield for wound dressings, even into the 20th century, and are used as tincture, cream or salve for skin wounds, infections and irritation, and control infection, bleeding and pain after burns and in radiation dermatitis. The tincture can also be taken internally for abdominal cramping and constipation, and an extract has been shown to have antitumor effects in laboratory animals. There are no major adverse effects, but allergic reactions may occur and the plant is best avoided during pregnancy.

Cascara *(Rhamnus purshiana)* is buckthorn or bearberry, a shrub native to western North America and used medicinally first by native Americans and then by Europeans. The bark contains hydroanthracene glycosides, which stimulate peristalsis of rhythmic contraction of the intestinal musculature, as well as the resin emodin, which causes smooth muscle cells to contract vigorously. The result is a powerful stimulant laxative, used since ancient times but named "sacred bark" *(cascara sagrada)* by Spanish explorers in the 17th century, and after its commercial introduction by the Parke-Davis company in 1877 the most commonly used pharmaceutical in North America and perhaps the most widely used drug in the world. The FDA banned the use of cascara and aloe in over-the-counter drug products in 2002 because of concerns about the development of tolerance and dependence, bleeding with prolonged use, abdominal pain and cramping, nausea and vomiting, loss of electrolytes and fluid through the gut, pigmentation of the intestines with long-term use *(melanosis coli)* and colon or rectal cancer. Cascara is still available as a herbal preparation, but should not be used for more than 7 days a time and ought to be taken with the guidance of an herbalist or physician.

Catnip *(Nepeta cataria)* is familiar to almost everyone but not usually thought of as a medicine for people. It is a member of the mint family related to marjoram, thyme, rosemary, sage and many other culinary spices, and contains nepetalactone, which repels flies, mosquitoes and roaches but attracts cats. It has a calming effect on humans, particularly colicky infants, and has also been used for fever and as a digestive aid. The leaves and flowers can be used in a calming tea, or a few drops of tincture can be used for infant colic. No adverse effects have been noted.

Cayenne *(Capsicum frutescens)* is a hot chili pepper in the nightshade family *(Solanaceae)* that is well-known in cooking and was described by Nicholas Culpeper in his 1653 herbal treatise as "Guinea pepper", a misnomer for Guiana in the Western Hemisphere, where it was first found. The pepper is high in vitamins A, B_2 (riboflavin), B_6, C and E, as well as manganese and potassium, but its chief medicinal ingredient is capsaicin, a volatile and very irritating compound that protects the plant from being eaten. Capsaicin dilates blood vessels, increases metabolic rate, enhances blood flow, regulates carbohydrate breakdown and insulin release, depletes the pain-initiating transmitter substance P and temporarily inactivates pain-sensing nerve cells with an influx of calcium. It is therefore effective against pain and FDA-approved for pharmaceutical use as an analgesic, and has been recommended as a supplement for circulatory insufficiency, diabetes and psoriasis. It is widely used in herbal practice for colds and sore throats, and as a cardiovascular tonic. There is some evidence that cayenne pepper is effective for addiction, cancer, heart disease, impotence, stroke and weight management, but this has not yet been substantiated. The fruit is most commonly dried and ground to make a topical ointment or tincture, and capsules are also available but can cause digestive upset. It is important to avoid eye contact with the fruit, seeds or medicinal preparation.

Chamomile is the name for several plants in the daisy family, of which the best known are *Matricaria chamomilla* (German chamomile) and *Chamamaelum nobile* (Roman, Russian or English chamomile). The name derives from the Greek and French for "earth apple", and these plants generally grow on the ground and are noteworthy because they grow more when they are trampled on. They contain many biologically active compounds, including the terpenes and lactones that are in many medicinal plants, coumarins that have anticoagulant effects and flavonoids that are effective antioxidants. There are also compounds that bind to receptors for the neurotransmitter *gamma*-aminbutyric acid (GABA) and regulate some other neurotransmitters, chiefly serotonin, as well as anti-inflammatory and hormone-like compounds. This makes them potentially useful for many disorders, and the chamomiles have traditionally been used for nervous and digestive disorders. The flowers can be made into teas, tinctures or capsules, and are usually used for anxiety, colic, diarrhea, eczema, gum inflammation and pain, heartburn and other forms of indigestion, inflammatory bowel diseases, insomnia, nervousness of various kinds and ulcers. The tincture can be applied to irritated or inflamed skin as an emollient, and chamomile will enhance the color of blonde hair. Some people are allergic to the flowers, and chamomile may interact with some drugs, particularly aspirin and blood thinners.

Cinnamon *(Cinnamomum zeylanicum)* is a spice obtained from the bark of several kinds of trees in the genus

Cinnamomum, which are part of the Laurel family *(Lauraceae)*. The trees are native to Ceylon and India, and the spice is mentioned in Egyptian papyri, the Hebrew Bible and the writings of the ancient Greeks. Cinnamon is widely used in cooking and fragrance, and is also an aromatherapy ingredient, fish and meat preservative and potentially an insect repellent. It has been felt to have warm and dry energy, and has been used in several traditional medical systems for infections, kidney disorders, skin conditions and snakebite among other problems, but some of its aromatic components, particularly coumarin, can cause liver damage in sensitive people. The inner bark is generally used as food, tincture or tea, or can be compounded into capsules. The warming energy of cinnamon makes it an effective circulatory tonic, and various kinds of bleeding disorders, colds and other respiratory infections, diarrhea and other digestive problems and menstrual bleeding are frequent indications for its use. An extract of cinnamon has been shown to inhibit the growth of several viruses, including herpes and HIV. Several of the flavonoids in cinnamon enhance insulin release and effect, and cinnamon extract may improve improve control in type 2 diabetes. Its antioxidant effect has been shown in several animal models to be protective against the development of melanoma and colorectal cancer, and there is also animal data that cinnamon inhibits the development of brain changes similar to those of Alzheimer's disease. Cinnamon is an ingredient in the beauty masks traditionally worn in some Asian cultures to improve complexion and eliminate acne and pimples. The main toxic concern is the effect of coumarin on the liver, either with high doses or pre-existing liver problems.

Clove *(Syzygium aromaticum)* is another spice of east Asian origin, derived from flower buds of an evergreen tree in the myrtle family *(Myrtaceae)*. Its strong aroma is due to the essential oil eugenol, and it is used in Asian, African and Middle Eastern cooking as well as the cuisine of Mexico, and to flavor cigars and cigarettes. Indian Ayurvedic and traditional Chinese medicine have long used clove: the Chinese call it *ding xiang* and consider it acrid, warm and aromatic, affecting the stomach, spleen and kidney meridians, warming the midsection and redirecting stomach *qi* downward and fortifying the *yang* of the kidney, while in the Indian tradition it is used for infections and as an antispasmodic. Western herbalism has used it as a carminative, to increase stomach acid and aid contraction, and as an antihelminthic to kill and expel worms. Eastern and western dentistry early recognized that it was an anodyne, and clove has long been applied to painful cavities and diseased teeth, as well as placed topically on the stomach and abdomen for pain and cramping. Essential oil from the buds is now most widely used, applying 1 or 2 drops to the gums for teething or onto painful teeth, being careful not to cause irritation of the mucous membranes with the oil.

Comfrey *(Symphytum officinalis)* was once called "knitbone" and the genus to which it belongs comes from the Greek for "plant" and "bones growing together". It was widely used to heal fractures and other injuries, but is now restricted to external use because of the demonstration that some of the alkaloids it contains are toxic to the liver and others may cause cancer. The ground root is made into a poultice and applied to skin lesions, areas of irritation, burns and the skin over sprains and fractures, where its chief beneficial ingredient, glyoxyldiureide or allantoin, can stimulate the growth of skin and possibly bone cells. The FDA has prohibited the internal use of comfrey, and it should not be applied for more than 10 days at a time or used more than 4 to 6 times a year.

Cornsilk *(Zea mays)* was first cultivated by the Aztecs and Mayas, who apparently prepared medicinal teas with it as early as 5000 BCE. It is rich in vitamins C and K, and contains a lot of potassium as well as antioxidant flavonoids and polyphenols, as well as demulcent compounds that soothe inflamed mucous membranes. Some people are allergic to corn and will react to the silk, and it should not be taken internally because toxic alkaloids are also present. It is widely used as a urinary tract tonic, and alleviates the irritable symptoms of cystitis or urinary tract infection as well as helping with bedwetting and perhaps hyperactive bladder.

Corydalis *(Corydalis turchaninovii* or *yanhusuo)* is named for the crested lark, a bird which it resembles, and the name covers a number of perennial or annual herbaceous plants (plants that have no woody stems above ground level) in the poppy family *(Papaveraceae)*. They grow in temperate zones of the Northern Hemisphere, are food for many species of butterflies and contain bulbocapnine, which inhibits the enzymes tyrosine hydroxylase, responsible for the metabolism of dopamine, and acetylcholinesterase, which breaks down acetylcholine, and is therefore a potent poison. The rhizome can be safely taken as a tincture or capsule, and is effective for insomnia and pain, especially menstrual. Fatigue, nausea and vomiting are occasional side effects, and pregnant and nursing women should avoid it because of the risks from even small amounts of the toxic alkaloid bulbocapnine.

Cranberry *(Vaccinium macrocarpon)* is widely considered a "superfruit" because of its high nutrient and antioxidant content. It is widely distributed in temperate parts of the Northern Hemisphere, but is chiefly cultivated in the United States and Canada. Polyphenol antioxidants, various chemicals that have cardiac and immune benefits as well as apparent anti-cancer activity, compounds that inhibit tooth decay and retard the formation of kidney stones and tannins that may slow blood clotting and prevent the adhesion of bacteria to the bladder and urethra in urinary tract infections, as well as high levels of many vitamins and trace minerals, have led to the widespread medicinal use of cranberry juice or extracts of the ripe fruit in capsule form. It is a mainstay of natural treatment of urinary tract infections, and has no significant adverse effects, although diabetics should be careful about the sugar content of its juice.

Damiana *(Turnera diffusa)* is a shrub native to the Southwestern United States, Mexico and the Caribbean, that has long been reputed to be an aphrodisiac. It does inhibit aromatase, an enzyme involved in metabolism of testosterone and estrogen, and can increase sexual behavior in animals. It contains several tannins, pigments and oils that may have anti-cancer effects, and has been used to make synthetic cannabis in the United States and the stimulant "Black Mamba" in the United Kingdom, in consequence of which Damiana has been banned in Britain and Louisiana. The leaves can be made into teas and tinctures or compounded as capsules or tablets, and have been used for depression, erectile dysfunction and low libido. Large amounts can cause diarrhea, and it should be avoided during pregnancy.

Dandelion *(Taraxacum officinale)* takes its name from the French *dent de lion* or "lion's tooth", referring to the jagged yellow petals of its flower. Dandelions evolved about 30 million years ago in Eurasia, and have been used as medicine and food throughout recorded history. Its powerful diuretic effect has long been known, and in most European languages the plant has a common name reflecting this (*e.g., piss-a-bed* in English, *pisse au lit* in French or *meacamas* in Spanish). Its greens are used in salad, its petals can be made into wine or ale, its flowers have been mixed with honey and made into jam and the ground roots will make a caffeine-free coffee. It is a mild laxative as well as a diuretic, stimulates gallbladder and liver function, is a general digestive tonic and has an emollient effect on the skin, as well as being a mosquito repellent and a folk remedy for warts. The root and leaf can be used in teas and tinctures or as capsules or tablets, but it can cause diarrhea and should be avoided with gallstones.

Devil's claw *(Harpagophytum procumbens)* is an African member of the sesame family with claw-shaped fruit that has long been used to treat pain and inflammation. The roots contain harpagoside, which is an effective anti-inflammatory compound but also interferes with blood clotting and increases the production of stomach acid. These effects warrant caution in people taking anticoagulants or with gallstones, ulcers or gastritis. The ground roots can otherwise be used as tincture, capsules or tablets for pain, particularly back pain, and inflammation, particularly arthritis, and also for digestive upset and indigestion.

Dong quai *(Angelica sinensis)* or "female ginseng" is a Chinese member of the carrot and parsley family *(Apiaceae)* that has been a mainstay of traditional Chinese medicine, used for anemia, fatigue, gynecological problems and high blood pressure. It is high in antioxidants and has steroid-like phytosterols, polysaccharides that enhance glucose metabolism and aromatic coumarins that lessen platelet adhesion and clot formation. It contains some potentially cancer-causing compounds and can cause skin photosensitivity, so high doses and use when pregnant or nursing should be avoided. The current herbalist use is tinctures, capsules or tablets made from the roots for anemia and pain due to menses as well as premenstrual syndrome and the symptoms of menopause.

Echinacea *(Echinacea purpurea* or *angustifolia)* or coneflower is a North American member of the daisy family that that has been used as a natural antibiotic. Some studies indicate that its roots and flowers enhance the response of the immune system and prevent or lessen bacterial, fungal or viral infections, but not all studies have confirmed this. There have also been suggestions that Echinacea can decrease the likelihood of getting various cancers and lessen the effects of chemotherapy and radiation treatments, but these have not yet been shown in controlled studies. The plant does contain fat-soluble alkylamides that may help to regulate cell migration, apoptosis or programmed cell death and the activation of tumor necrosis factor, effects that might contribute to cancer prevention, and many phenol compounds are present that can influence the immune system. The roots and flowers are usually used for teas, tinctures, capsules or tablets and can be taken to prevent colds and flu or to shorten their duration and lessen their severity. People with autoimmune disorders should not use this on a long-term basis, and those who are allergic to daisies should avoid Echinacea.

Elderberry *(Sambucus nigra)* is a group of several flowering shrubs related to the honeysuckle, and grows in the temperate parts of the Americas and Australia. The tree was thought in some places to ward off evil but in other areas to be a congregating place for witches. Its flowers and berries are used to make wine and flavor liquors, and in some countries for soft drinks, as well as jams and desserts. They are dissolved in wine and used for rheumatism and pain after trauma by Chinese herbalists. The uncooked berries are poisonous, because one of the glycosides in them is metabolized to cyanide, but the cooked berries are safe, and an extract of them has been shown to increase cytokine production and protect against influenza and the common cold. Tinctures and teas have been used after cold or flu exposure or at the onset of symptoms, and commercially available syrups are effective with few adverse effects.

Eyebright *(Euphrasia officinalis)* gets its name from a long tradition of use for eye diseases, particularly conjunctivitis. Eyebright is actually a genus of some 450 herbaceous flowering plants that grow in mountain regions. Its medicinal use was known to the Greeks and Romans but lost until the Middle Ages, when it was rediscovered by oculists and apothecaries; Culpeper associated it with the zodiac sign Leo, and recommended it for memory problems and vertigo, but it has most often been used for eyestrain or eye infection. A poultice of the whole herb was formerly applied around the eye, but a tincture is now usually used as an eyewash or capsules taken orally. Allergies affecting the eye, conjunctivitis ("pink eye"), and cough, congestion and eye irritation from sinus problems are the usual indications, and side effects are essentially nil.

Fennel *(Foeniculum vulgare)* is a flowering plant related to celery that is native to the Mediterranean area but is now widely grown and commonly used in cooking. *Foeniculum* is the diminutive of *faenum*, Latin for "hay", which the plant resembles. The stalk of the fennel plant was what Prometheus used to steal fire from the demigods, and Dionysus and his followers made wands for their wild parties, or bacchanalia, from the giant fennel plant. Funchal, the capital of Portugal's Madeira islands, was named for the fennel that grew everywhere on the island. The aromatic compound anethole is responsible for the smell and flavor of the plant, and is very similar to camphor, while the plant also contains estrogen-like compounds. The seeds are for this reason used for menstrual pain and to increase breast milk production, as well as for colic and intestinal gas, and like camphor, it can be used for cough and respiratory congestion. It can be applied to the chest or taken internally as a tincture, or made into capsules with no major adverse effects.

Fenugreek *(Trigonella foenumgraecum)* was cultivated by the Egyptians and in ancient India, and was known to the Greeks and Romans. The seeds and leaves have a characteristic sweet smell due to the lactone sotolon, and are used in Indian curries and pickles, Middle Eastern salads and the breads of Egypt and Ethiopia. Its main medicinal use is for diabetes, and it enhances insulin release and facilitates the absorption of glucose by cells as well as lowering cholesterol levels and being a digestive tract tonic and demulcent. The seeds are generally ground and used for tinctures or teas. It is important to make sure that imported seeds have been screened for bacterial contamination by *E. coli,* as these were linked to an outbreak of disease in Europe in 2011.

Feverfew *(Tenacetum parthenium)* is a perennial plant in the daisy family, sometimes called "bachelor's button" because it has been worn by wedding parties. Its name came from "fever reducer", which it was once thought to be, but the plant has been used for inflammation since Dioscorides described it in the 1st century. Its active ingredients, the lactone parthenolide and the terpene tanetin, have been shown to reduce the inflammation that is one of the triggers of migraine as well as a factor in various kinds of arthritis, and to activate programmed cell death and inactivate stem cells that can develop into tumors in some animal models of cancer. The leaves are used for tinctures or made into capsules, and can cause contact dermatitis or mouth ulcers if applied directly, as well as occasional nausea, vomiting and flatulence. Feverfew can also interact with blood thinners and some drugs metabolized by the cytochrome P450 system in the liver and cause bleeding and side effects. It is not recommended for children under 2 years old or for pregnant or nursing women. Not all brands of feverfew have specified how much parthenolide they contain and some studies have shown great variability between brands; the effective parthenolide dose for inflammation and migraine is about 0.2 to 0.6 mg, and a standardized parthenolide content of 0.7 per cent is recommended.

Flax seeds *(Linum usitatissimum)*, known as common flax or linseed, is a fiber crop grown in cooler regions around the world. It is one of the oldest domesticated plants, and was cultivated as long as 30,000 years ago. It has been used to make linen since the Neolithic period, and was used by the Greeks and Romans for sails as well. The health benefits of linseed oil were known to the ancients and advocated by Charlemagne among others. It is now generally grown for nutrition, wood finishing and as a garden ornament, and still justifies its Latin name, which means "most useful". The seeds contain lignans, phenol compounds that are antioxidants, have estrogen-like effects and may reduce tumor growth, as well as high levels of fiber, many micronutrients and *omega*-3 fatty acids. Powdered seeds or oil can be directly applied to the skin as an emollient and a source of fatty acids for dryness or inflammation, or the oil or seeds can be taken internally as a fiber supplement, laxative and anti-inflammatory, with diarrhea from excessive doses the chief caution.

Garlic *(Allium sativa)* has been used by humans for over 7,000 years, first in its native central Asia and now worldwide. There are two main subspecies of garlic, 10 major groups of garlic varieties and hundreds of cultivars or varieties, chiefly soft-necked (sativum) and hard-necked (ophioscoridon). Almost all of the plant is edible and it is used in almost every culture. The first Chinese medical textbooks from around 2000 BCE mention its use, as do the writings of Hippocrates 1500 years later, and modern studies have confirmed or suggested its benefit for elevated cholesterol and blood sugar, high blood pressure, heart disease, complications of diabetes, bacterial and fungal infection, scurvy and beriberi, low testosterone, gangrene, tooth decay, infections related to HIV and AIDS and possibly even the common cold. Allicin and the other sulfur-containing compounds that give garlic its pungency, which serve to protect the plant against pest attack, appear to be responsible for these potential benefits also. Fresh garlic cloves or dried and ground cloves in tinctures, tea, tablets or capsules are currently recommended for immune support, high cholesterol, cardiac protection and cancer prevention, and eardrops are effective against ear infection and pain. It can cause digestive upset and in its fresh forms can affect the breath.

Gentian *(Gentiana lutea)* refers to a large genus of plants containing around 450 species, characterized by large trumpet-shaped flowers that are intensely blue in color. They are named for Gentius, who in the 2nd century BCE ruled Illyria, which is present-day Albania, and who is said to have discovered the tonic properties of the herb. It gives a bitter flavor to aperitifs, liquers and tonics, and has long been used for the herbal treatment of digestive disorders, fever, malaria, parasitic infections, muscle spasms and high blood pressure, and is reputed to be effective for cancer. Gentian violet is a vivid dye made from the leaves, and a 1 per cent solution can be applied to areas of thrush or *Candida* infection in the mouth, but should not be swallowed. The dye can also be used as a disinfectant and for skin infections such as ringworm or athlete's foot. A tincture or capsules prepared from the ground root can be taken for malabsorption and poor appetite, particularly as part of a chronic illness, but can aggravate heartburn, gastritis or ulcers.

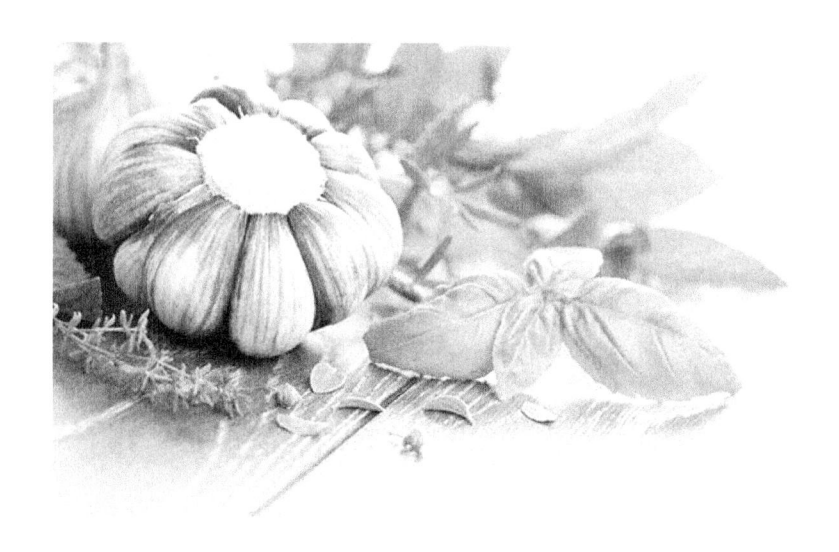

Ginger *(Zingiber officinalis)* was originally cultivated in Southwest Asia, and became the basis of the ancient spice trade because it was used for cooking, medicine and as a delicacy from earliest recorded history. It is crucial to Chinese, Japanese and Korean cooking, is used in sauces in Indian cuisine and is used as a flavoring, particularly for beverages, in the Middle East and in the West. Indian Ayurvedic medicine advocates eating ginger with each meal as a digestive tonic, and uses it for pain, menstrual and other types of bleeding, dizziness and vertigo and inflammation as well as a digestive tonic. Traditional Chinese medicine uses the intense warming energy of ginger oil, raw or powdered ginger and combination herbal preparations including ginger for allergies, arthritis, atherosclerosis, coughs and colds, morning sickness, nausea and vomiting, respiratory infections and congestion and side effects of cancer chemotherapy. Western herbal practice uses the ground roots in tea, tincture or capsules for digestive symptoms, poor appetite and particularly for gas, as well as for inflammation, alleviation of sore throat and prevention of colds.

Ginkgo *(Ginkgo biloba)* is the national tree of China and is a living fossil, dating back 270 million years and similar to many ancient ferns but with no living relatives. Ginkgo trees are extraordinarily resistant to insects, plant diseases and weather, and some have been estimated to be 2500 or more years old; 6 ginkgo trees at the epicenter of the Hiroshima atomic bomb blast were the only living things to survive and are growing there still. The tree has fan-shaped leaves divided into two lobes ("biloba"), an arrangement that is unique among seed plants, and has long been revered by Buddhists and followers of Confucius, frequently grown as *bonsai* and the symbol of the Japanese tea ceremony. The nut-like seed pods are reputed to be aphrodisiacs and are used in the Chinese *congee* rice porridge as well as the vegetarian Buddha's delight often served at the New Year, but also contain an inhibitor of vitamin B_6 (pyridoxine) that can cause convulsions if eaten in large amounts of by small children. The leaves are safer, and contain flavonoids such as myrecetin and quercitin, as well as terpenes like ginkgolides and bilobalide, which are potent antioxidants, inhibit the reuptake of several neurotransmitters and inhibit the aggregation of platelets and slow blood clotting. Tinctures or capsules prepared from the leaf are widely used in natural medicine, with some evidence of effectiveness for attention deficit disorder, cataracts, dementia, depression, high blood pressure, impotence, macular degeneration, memory problems, Meniere's disease and other tinnitus and vertigo, migraine, peripheral vascular disease, premenstrual syndrome, radiation toxicity, Raynaud's disease, retinopathy from diabetes and other diseases and stroke prevention and recovery. The chief benefits have been in cognitive improvement in dementia, although ginkgo does not prevent the onset of Alzheimer's disease, and in improvement of circulation, although bleeding must be watched for in those also taking aspirin or anticoagulants and headache and digestive upset may also occur, while some people are sensitive to the skin-irritating effect of the leaves and should not handle them. Because ginkgo can elevate brain levels of dopamine, norpinephrine and serotonin, it should not be combined with SSRI (selective serotonin-reuptake inhibiting), SNRI (selective norepinephine and serotonin-reuptake inhibiting) and MAOI (monoamine oxidase inhibiting) antidepressants.

Ginseng refers to 3 different plants, the *Chinese (Panax ginseng)*, *Siberian (Eleutherococcus senticosus)* and *American (Panax quinquefolia)* varieties, which are members of the ivy family (*Araliaceae*). These were first described by 17th-century Jesuit missionaries in China, who brought them back to Europe, and have been recognized in Eastern and Western herbal medicine as adaptogens, stimulants and aphrodisiacs. The whole or sliced dried root has been used in traditional Chinese medicine, and Western herbal medicine uses dried and ground root for tinctures or teas and in capsules. Chinese ginseng is warming, while the energy of Siberian and American ginseng is cooling. These roots, particularly the *Panax* species, contain ginsenosides as well as estrogen-like compounds, and have been shown to increase white blood cell count and the number of "cytotoxic" and "natural killer" T cell lymphocytes that are involved in immune defense against viruses and cancer cells. Reduction in the number and severity of herpes outbreaks in people infected with the viruses has been shown with Siberian ginseng, and asthma has been treated with American ginseng. The main medicinal use of the ginsengs is to counteract stress and lessen physical, mental and emotional fatigue. Chinese ginseng can cause overstimulation and may precipitate mania in depressed patients taking antidepressants, and can lower blood alcohol levels but not necessarily alleviate intoxication. Insomnia, nosebleeds, increased or decreased blood pressure, nausea, diarrhea and headache are also possible side effects.

Goldenseal *(Hydrastis canadensis)*, sometimes called orangeroot or yellow puccoon, is a relative of the buttercup that has many medicinal properties: it is at once an alterative, anticatarrhal, anti-inflammatory, antimicrobial, astringent, bitter, cholagogue, emmenagogue, hepatic, laxative, oxytocic and stimulant. It is widely used in herbalism, often to enhance the effects of other herbal medicines. Native Americans used it as a digestive tonic, eyewash and cancer treatment, and it became a mainstay of the American Eclectic school of natural medicine in the 19th century. More than 20 alkaloids have been isolated from the plant, chiefly berberine and hydrastine, which are potent antimicrobials and also inhibit the ability of bacteria to develop antibiotic resistance. It is highly cooling, and has been advocated for fever but not for chills, and inhibits the cytochrome systems in the liver, which metabolize many drugs, so should not be combined with many pharmaceutical drugs, particularly SSRI antidepressants, neuroleptics and codeine. The herb has been reputed to simulate the presence of poisons such as strychnine and drugs of abuse such as morphine in urine toxicology tests, but this has not been confirmed. There has also been concern about the toxic effects of berberine, which is present in several other plants (Oregon grape, philodendron, coptis, barberry and yellowroot) as well as goldenseal, and berberine-containing herbal preparations are considered potentially hazardous by the drug regulators of the European Union. American agencies and practitioners recommend that goldenseal and other berberine-containing herbs not be used for more than 2 weeks and not by pregnant or nursing women, and that the herb be stopped if digestive upset occurs. Tinctures or capsules prepared from the roots have been used for infections or irritation of the mucous membranes, colds and flu, digestive problems including diarrhea and parasitic infections. Another problem with goldenseal is that the plant is endangered in some places due to overharvesting and habitat destruction, and some of the above-mentioned plants that also contain berberine may be appropriate alternatives.

Gotu Kola *(Centella asiatica)*, the African or Indian pennywort, has long been used in the traditional medicine of Africa, China and India. It is related to carrot and parsley and grows in ditches and wet lowlands. It is widely used in Indian, Sri Lankan, Malay, Vietnamese and Thai cooking, and is used for many illnesses, chiefly memory problems, in Ayurvedic practice. Gotu kola was thought to be responsible for the longevity of the herbalist and *tai chi* master Li Ching-Yuen, who died in 1933 at what was widely believed in China to be the age of either 197 or 256 years. Anecdotal reports of cancer remission with gotu kola have not been accepted by the American Cancer Society, but it has been shown as one of the constituents of the combination herbal preparation Pycnogenol to reverse the progression of carotid and femoral artery occlusive disease in patients who did not yet have symptoms of circulatory insufficiency or stroke. The roots and leaves are usually used to make tinctures and capsules, and it has been used to reduce scar formation after burns and skin injury, to facilitate the healing of connective tissue, to improve memory and to reduce lung and lymph node inflammation in sarcoidosis.

Green Tea *(Camellia sinensis)* is made from tea leaves that have undergone minimal oxidation during processing, and is a staple of Asian cultures but has only recently been widely consumed in the West, where black tea has historically been preferred. The health benefits of green tea were known in China as early as the second millennium BCE, and the *Tea Classic* of Lu Yu, written between 600 and 900 A.D., prescribes the manner of making tea for health as well as pleasure; the Japanese *Book of Tea*, written around 1191 by the priest Eisai, who introduced both green tea and Zen into Japan, summarizes the effects of tea on the five vital organs, particularly the heart. The eastern herbal traditions hold that tea lessens the effects of alcohol, functions as a stimulant, quenches thirst, eliminates indigestion, lessens fatigue and forestalls beriberi. The flavonoid content of a cup of green tea is higher than an equivalent volume of almost any other fruit, vegetable or drink, which makes it a potent antioxidant, while the combination of phenols and caffeine increases metabolic rate without increasing heart rate, so may assist with weight loss. Green tea consumption is associated with decreased risk of heart disease, Alzheimer's disease, Parkinson's disease and some cancers, and total cholesterol and LDL cholesterol are reduced by regular drinking of green tea. It is also recommended as a digestive tonic and detoxifying agent, and can reduce or prevent tooth decay. Insomnia and anxiety are the main adverse effects, and these can be avoided by using green tea capsules or tincture of tea leaves.

Guggul *(Comiphora wightii)* is the Indian form of myrrh, a member of the family to which the frankincense and myrrh of the Bible belong (*Bursuraceae*). It is an important medical plant in the Ayurvedic tradition, but its availability and use are now limited because the species is endangered due to overuse. The resinous sap of the plant, known as gum guggul, produces a useful extract (guggulipid) that contains a compound (guggulsterone) that may beneficially affect cholesterol metabolism, although there have also been studies questioning its usefulness for prevention of atherosclerosis. Capsules and tablets containing the gum have also been used for hypothyroidism, but guggul should be avoided during pregnancy and when breastfeeding and digestive upset need to be watched for.

Gymnema *(Gymnema sylvestre)* is another Indian herb long used in Ayurvedic medicine, and is one of the chief natural remedies for diabetes. The major active constituents are saponins, large soap-like organic molecules grouped together as gymnemic acids, which reduce sweet taste on the tongue by blocking the receptors for sweet taste on the tongue, as well as enhancing insulin secretion in animal models and human type 2 diabetes, potentially reversing insulin resistance and apparently regenerating or repairing insulin-secreting pancreatic cells. Some patients with type 2 diabetes and insulin resistance were able to discontinue pharmaceutical drugs and have adequate glucose control; if confirmed in larger studies, this may confirm gymnema's title in Indian traditional medicine of "miracle fruit". Tinctures, tablets and capsules are made from the leaves, and have no significant side effects, although it is recommended to avoid gymnema when pregnant or breastfeeding.

Hawthorn *(Crataegus oxycantha)* is sometimes called thornapple or hawberry and is a member of the rose family along with most of the edible fruits, almonds and the roses and other ornamental bushes. The tart red berries are widely used in cooking in both eastern and western cultures, and healing traditions in several cultures have used the berries medicinally, chiefly for cardiovascular disease. Tannins, flavonoids and phenols are active ingredients capable of retarding or reversing heart disease, and large studies have generally but not always shown that hawthorn extract reduces the incidence and severity of heart failure, lessens the risk of arrhythmia and improves blood pressure, measures of cardiac function and exercise tolerance. The berries are used to make tinctures, tablets and capsules, and adverse effects are few but there can be interactions with digitalis and other heart medications.

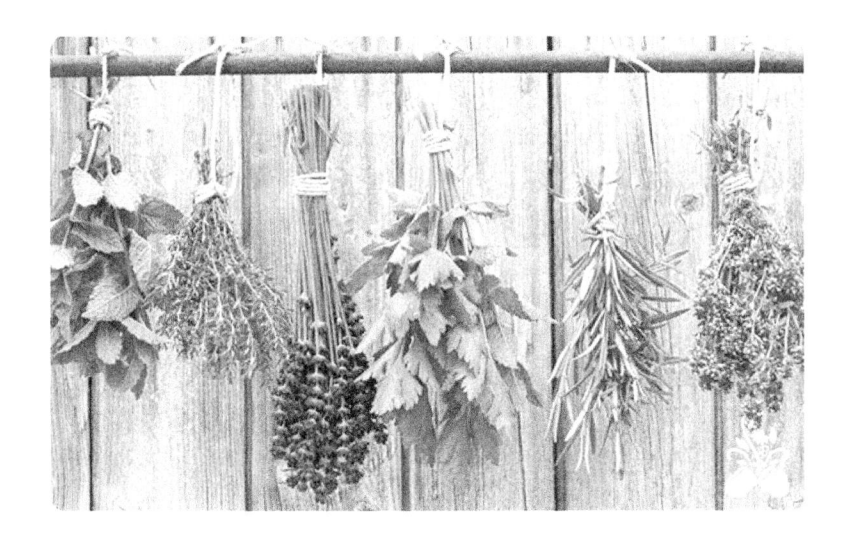

Hops *(Humulus lupulus)* have been cultivated in Europe since the 8th century, and began to be used in brewing about 200 years later. The plant was introduced to the New World in the 17th century. The major use of the female flowers of the plant is in beer, but nonalcoholic beverages are also made in Europe, Latin America and Russia. The medicinal uses of hops have chiefly been for restlessness, anxiety and insomnia, and a pillow full of hops is a traditional sleep aid; hops have more recently attracted attention for menstrual disturbances and hormonal replacement because they contain plant estrogen compounds (phytoestrogens). The fruiting bodies or strobile are used for tinctures, teas and capsules, and are recommended for anxiety, sleep problems and digestive symptoms like stomach pain and colic, with no significant side effects noted.

Horehound *(Marrubium vulgaris)* is a European perennial plant in the family that includes mint, rosemary, sage, thyme, marjoram and oregano. It has been used medicinally since Roman times, chiefly for respiratory ailments. The first *Herball*, published by John Gerard in 1597, recommended it for respiratory congestion and to expel worms. The essential oil of the flowers has anticancer and antiseptic properties, and its main ingredient, marrubin, is an anti-inflammatory compound that reverses atherosclerosis and improves diabetes. Horehound has long been used to make lozenges for cough and respiratory mucus, and has been recommended in tincture form for asthma. There are no significant adverse effects.

Horse chestnut *(Aesculus hippocastum)* is a tree native to the Balkans, but is now distributed worldwide. The name is doubly wrong, because the tree is not in the chestnut family and the fruit, once thought to cure horses of chest disorders, is in fact poisonous to them. The nuts, especially fresh ones, are mildly poisonous to humans but the seeds contain aescin, a saponin that strengthens blood vessel walls, apparently by increasing nitric oxide synthesis by their endothelial cells. Aescin is also mildly anti-inflammatory, and may enhance the health of endothelial cells by slowing the breakdown of cell wall components. Whereas much of the evidence supporting herbal medicines is anecdotal, there are controlled trials that suggest that horse chestnut extract is more effective for venous insufficiency than compression stockings. Tinctures, tablets and capsules containing the extract are used for varicose veins, hemorrhoids and back pain, and the main problems involve occasional headache, digestive upset and itching.

Horsetail *(Equisetum arvense)* is the last survivor of the *Equisetaceae*, flowering plants that reproduced by spores and once dominated the forests of the Paleozoic era 200 to 600 million years ago. The leaves are grouped around nodes, which are closer together toward the apex of the plant and resemble a horse's tail, and it is said that this geometric pattern gave the Scottish botanist and mathematician John Napier the idea for logarithms around 1600. Extracts of the plant contain an enzyme not found anywhere else in the plant kingdom, which apparently stops the growth of cells during their aging process. This might make the horsetail medically useful, but there are also small amounts of nicotine and an enzyme that breaks down thiamine (vitamin B_1), so caution is appropriate in its use. The South American variant of the plant is widely used as a diuretic and for urinary tract infections, and contains silicon, which may help preserve bone strength. European studies suggest that horsetail may help skin, bone and hair health, restore general vigor and facilitate weight loss. The main herbal use presently of tinctures, teas and capsules made from the plant's stem is for urinary tract infections and as a silica supplement, and no significant adverse effects are reported.

Huperzia *(Huperzia serrata)* is a club moss called *qian ceng ta* or *jin bu huan* by the Chinese, found as about 400 different species around the world and widely sold as a nootropic agent and a dietary supplement to enhance memory and improve brain function. The basis of this effect is huperizine A, which inhibits acetylcholinesterase, which breaks down the memory and neuromuscular transmitter acetylcholine, and blocks the NMDA (*N*-methyl-*d*-aspartate) receptor that is involved in neurodegenerative disorders. This is what pharmaceutical drugs for Alzheimer's disease do, and there is some evidence that huperizine A is also effective for dementia. The moss is dried and ground for tablets and capsules, and has no adverse effects except possibly interacting with other medications that affect acetylcholine metabolism, either in the central nervous system or at the neuromuscular junction.

Kava or **kava-kava** *(Piper methysticum)* is a South Pacific relative of common black pepper whose Latin name means "intoxicating pepper". It has been used in Hawaii, Polynesia, Micronesia and Melanesia to promote relaxation and calm without affecting mental clarity, and it has been suggested that Aldous Huxley had it in mind when he wrote about *soma* in the novel *Brave New World*. At least 15 kavalactones have been isolated from the plant and have psychoactive effects, possibly increasing norepinephrine and GABA levels to produce euphoria and enhanced mental clarity, but not affecting serotonin or dopamine levels to produce mood changes or sedation. These lactones may also act on cannabinoid receptors, which are responsible for some of the psychic effects of marijuana. A very rigorous review of clinical trials has suggested that kava-kava is better than placebo for the treatment of anxiety, but occasional liver toxicity and rare liver failure have led to the regulation of kava in some countries. It is recommended in western herbal medicine for anxiety, hyperactivity, insomnia and muscle spasms, using tinctures, teas or capsules prepared from the dried root, but should not be used by pregnant or breastfeeding women or those with liver problems, and should not be combined with alcohol use or prescription anxiety or antidepressant medication.

Lavender *(Lavendula augustifolia)* is a member of the mint family that has been cultivated since ancient times, and the name may be derived from the Latin term for "blue-tinged". The essential oil from the flowers has long been used as a fragrance, and has antiseptic and antimicrobial properties; the modern science of aromatherapy was born in 1910 when perfume chemist René Gattefossé burned his hand in a laboratory accident, dipped it in lavender oil because nothing else was handy and noticed that the burn healed. Infusions of lavender flowers are also used, and their effect may be due to the alcohol linalool, which is a precursor of vitamin E. Lavender oil capsules have been found as effective as lorazepam for anxiety in Germany, and applying small amounts of lavender oil or inhalation of lavender vapor help tension headaches as well as anxiety. It is also recommended for stress-related digestive problems, insomnia and muscle spasms and external use is preferable.

Lemon balm *(Melissa officinalis)* is a perennial herb in the mint family, and is not a lemon but smells like one. It is widely used as a flavoring ingredient, and was used in ancient times for gastrointestinal and nervous problems. Carmelite water, an alcohol extract of the herb and several others, was first prepared by nuns in the 14th century, and is still sold in Europe. The essential oil is widely used in aromatherapy, and tinctures or teas have been found effective for anxiety, work stress, low-dose radiation exposure and as a mosquito repellant. Lemon balm extract contains eugenol, terpenes and tannins that have antioxidant effects and also inhibit GABA transaminase and acetylcholinesterase, so lemon balm teas and tinctures can alleviate anxiety and possibly improve mental acuity and performance. These also prevent thyroid-stimulating hormone from attaching to its receptors, so lemon balm is appropriate treatment for hyperthyroid states such as Graves's disease but should be avoided by hypothyroid people. Other current herbal medicine uses are depression, fever, genital and oral herpes infections and respiratory tract infections, using tinctures or salves from the whole plant.

Licorice *(Glycorrhiza glabra)* means "sweet root", and its culinary and medicinal uses were summarized by Dioscorides in the 1st century. Anethole is responsible for its anise-like smell, and has antimicrobial and insecticidal effects but is also a major component of the potentially toxic liquor absinthe and an inexpensive precursor of illicit amphetamine derivatives. Glycyrrhizin is 30 to 50 times sweeter than sugar and is an anti-inflammatory compound that mimics the effects of adrenal gland hormones and is also effective against many viruses. Other components of the licorice root are estrogen-like. In traditional Chinese medicine, licorice is used to harmonize the ingredients in multi-herb presentations and to carry their effects to each of the 12 "regular" meridians that regulate organ functions. Western natural medicine has used it for mouth ulcers and peptic ulcer disease, with some indication that it can alleviate hepatitis, reduce elevated blood lipids, reverse tooth decay and lessen allergic dermatitis. The cortisol-like effects of licorice, causing edema, elevated potassium levels, weight gain and hypertension, have limited its medicinal use. Tinctures, teas, capsules and creams made from the root are recommended for adrenal gland support, asthma, chronic fatigue, cold sores, cough, digestive disorders, heartburn, hepatitis, immune system support, inflammatory conditions, liver support, muscle spasms, ulcers and shingles, as well as to increase the effectiveness of other herbs. High doses causing fluid retention should be avoided, and it is not recommended in pregnancy, breastfeeding or hypertension.

Lomatium *(Lomatium dissectum)* is a North American edible herb related to carrots and parsley, sometimes called Indian parsley because of its use for food and medicine by native Americans. It has historically been used for respiratory conditions, particularly tuberculosis, and an extract of the root has been shown to neutralize the effects of rotavirus and have antibiotic effect against tuberculosis bacilli. Tinctures or capsules made from the root are recommended for immune support, colds and flu and urinary tract infections, with caution for skin rash and avoidance during pregnancy because of its antibiotic effects.

Maitake *(Grifola frondosa)* is a mushroom that grows at the base of trees, especially oaks. It is known as "dancing mushroom" by Asians, called "signorina mushroom" by Italian-Americans and is often used in cooking by both. In eastern herbal medicine, it is used to balance or harmonize body systems and enhance the immune system. Western herbal research suggests that maitake activates natural killer cells for immune defense, enhances programmed cell death and inhibits the growth of cancer cells, lowers blood sugar, contains antioxidants and inhibits the inflammation-initiating enzyme cyclooxygenase. The fruiting body of the mushroom is dried and ground for tinctures and capsules that are recommended for general immune support, hepatitis, adjunctive therapy for cancer and HIV infection and better control of diabetes and high cholesterol. No significant side effects are reported.

Marshmallow *(Althea officinalis)* is not the widely-enjoyed sugar candy but rather an African perennial plant related to okra, cotton and cacao. The name of the genus comes from the Greek *althein,* "to heal", and marshmallow has been used since ancient times in China for bronchial inflammation and deficient flow of breast milk, while the extracted flowers have been used since the Middle Ages for sore throat. The root is used to make Middle Eastern *halva,* and in France was whipped into a meringue called *guimauve* or "marshmallow", which is now made commercially with sugar and does not contain the marshmallow plant. The root is highly soothing to mucous membranes as tincture or tea and in capsules or tablets, and is recommended for asthma, cough, diarrhea, inflammatory bowel disorders, respiratory infections, ulcers and urinary tract infections, with no known adverse effects.

Milk thistle *(Silybum marianum)* is a member of the daisy family sometimes called Scotch thistle or St. Mary's thistle. Originally from England, the plant got its identification with the Virgin Mary when it was grown in monastery gardens for food and medicinal use; it now grows worldwide and in many countries is considered a weed. Extracts of the seeds contain silymarin, which has properties of flavonoids and phenol compounds and is thus an effective antioxidant. This protects the liver against toxins, regenerates liver cells lost to various forms of liver damage, has a rejuvenating effect on the gallbladder and improves control of type 2 diabetes while helping to prevent the development of the metabolic syndrome of obesity, insulin resistance, abnormal blood lipids and hypertension. There is also evidence that silymarin may be effective for obsessions and compulsions, and in laboratory studies it inhibits some tumor cells and stimulates the growth of lymphocytes and nerve cells. Tinctures, capsules and tablets prepared from the seeds are recommended for addiction treatment, particularly alcoholism, constipation, gallstones, indigestion, protection of the liver and repair of liver damage, premenstrual syndrome and skin disorders, particularly acne and eczema. No specific side effects are reported.

Motherwort *(Leonurus cardiaca)* is a member of the mint family that derives its common name from a long history of obstetrical use by midwives. It is a uterine tonic and prevents uterine infection, as well as being a cardiac tonic, a relaxing nervine and functioning as an emmenagogue, due in part to flavonoids, tannins and vitamin A, and in part to the alkaloid leonurine, which dilates blood vessels and relaxes the smooth muscle of the uterus. Some western herbalists recommend it for stress relief and relaxation during pregnancy and prevention of hemorrhage during labor; others have suggested that it be avoided during pregnancy as it may cause bleeding and induce miscarriage. The Chinese call its leaves *yi mu cao* and consider them bitter and spicy in flavor and cold in energy, primarily affecting the bladder, heart and liver and useful to prevent pregnancy and regulate menstruation. Most natural practitioners use tinctures, teas, capsules or tablets made from leaves and flowers to reduce palpitations and anxiety due to menopause and to alleviate absent or abnormal menstrual periods, and do not use it during pregnancy.

Mullein *(Verbascum thapsis)* is a minimally aggressive weed that prefers to grow in soil that has been disturbed and is well lit. It has been used to make dyes, but also has a medicinal history dating back to ancient times. It has also been used to weaken fish so they can be caught, and has been suggested to be both an implement of witches and a means of warding off curses and spells. The Greeks and Romans used decoctions of boiled leaves or steeped teas for cough and pulmonary diseases, while Native Americans smoked the dried leaves or made syrups for consumption and croup. The leaves contain saponins which mobilize mucus as well as lubricating mucilage, so it has frequently been used for cough but also applied as a poultice for sores, rashes and skin infections. Oil from the flowers has been used for boils, chilblains, colic, earaches, eczema, frostbite, hemorrhoids and respiratory congestion, and has been found to contain glycyrrhizin as does licorice, making it a potential antibiotic. The German Commission E has endorsed its use for respiratory congestion, and tinctures, teas and capsules made from the leaves or topically-applied oil from the flowers are widely used for asthma, bronchitis, cough, chronic obstructive pulmonary disease, ear infections and upper respiratory infections, with no significant adverse effects.

Myrrh *(Commiphora myrrha)* is an oleoresin, an aromatic natural gum that is obtained from the bark of a thorny African and Arabian tree. Various members of the *Commiphora* genus produce myrrh, frankincense, Balm of Gilead, Balsam of Mecca and other ointments, incenses and chrisms described in ancient Egyptian papyri, the Talmud, various Islamic texts and the Christian Bible. Myrrh is also part of the Chinese medical tradition, considered bitter and spicy in flavor and neutral in temperature and used for the heart, liver and spleen, as well as to purge stagnant blood; myrrh is often used to move blood and frankincense to move *qi*, as well as being combined with other herbs, usually mixed in alcohol for external or internal use. The Indian Ayurvedic tradition calls myrrh *daindhava* and uses it in *rasayana* ("path of essence") formulas aimed at increasing longevity, while the Islamic Unani tradition often used myrrh by itself as a tonic and rejuvenating agent. Western herbalism uses myrrh as an antiseptic in mouthwash and toothpaste, as an analgesic for toothache and a liniment for bruises and sprains and as a veterinary tincture; myrrh has also been shown to lower blood sugar, lower total and "bad" cholesterol and increase "good" cholesterol levels and combat parasitic infection, as well as alleviating pain and inhibiting cancer growth in animal models. The principal herbal medicine use currently is treatment of throat and mouth infections with tincture of the resin, avoiding high doses internally because of the risk of diarrhea and kidney irritation.

Nettles *(Urtica dioica)* are sometimes called stinging nettles because of their needle-like hairs, which inject histamine, acetylcholine, serotonin and several other irritants on contact. Nettles grow in every American state and Canadian province except Hawaii, and are strongly associated with human habitation and buildings and possibly nourished by human and animal wastes. Nettles are cooked in various ways in many cultures, and there is an annual raw nettle-eating contest in Marshwood, Dorset in the United Kingdom. Nettle leaves and roots have traditionally been used for urinary tract and rheumatic disorders, as a galactogogue to promote lactation and as a counter-irritant for skin disorders and tonic to improve the glossiness of hair. Recent studies have shown that nettle leaf extracts reduce tumor necrosis factor-*alpha* and other cytokines that promote inflammation, and improve diabetic control by increasing insulin production and release. Nettle root extracts shrink hypertrophied prostate tissue and relieve symptoms of prostatism, and contain lignans that increase free testosterone levels with benefit in bodybuilding. Both leaves and roots are very high in mineral content. Tinctures, teas, salves and capsules are made from leaves or root, and are currently recommended for prostate enlargement (root) and anemia, arthritis, brittle hair, edema, hay fever, skin rash and general detoxification (leaves), with no major adverse effects.

Oatstraw *(Avena sativa)* is almost universally accepted as a healthy food, and is widely eaten by people and generally fed to animals. The outer casing (bran) lowers LDL cholesterol, and oats contain more soluble fiber than any other grain, which slows digestion and increases the sensation of satiety. Oats are also second only to corn in lipid content, and have a high level of protein comparable to soy protein. Oats are also free of most of the proteins that constitute gluten, and can be an alternative grain for most people unable to tolerate wheat on account of celiac disease or other gluten sensitivity. Another medicinal benefit from oats and oatstraw is through topical application as an oatmeal bath for itchy skin. Depression, fatigue, restlessness and stress may be alleviated by tea or tincture in water or on the tongue, or oatstraw can be taken in capsule form.

Oregano *(Origanum vulgare)* is a perennial herb in the mint family, originally grown around the Mediterranean but now used throughout the world. It has an aromatic, slightly bitter, warm taste that figures importantly in Mediterranean, Latin American and Philippine cooking. It has a high content of antioxidant flavonoids and phenols, and has antibacterial effects. It has long been used in Southern Europe and the Middle East for colds and sore throats, and in some parts of Central Europe for gastrointestinal, respiratory and nervous complaints. The leaves and dried herb, which is more potent than the fresh plant, are used to make tinctures and capsules, which are recommended particularly for fungal infections such as candidiasis. It has no especial adverse effects, but should be avoided during pregnancy.

Oregon grape *(Mahonia aquefolium)* is not a grape but its berries look like them; it is in fact an evergreen shrub with spiny holly-like leaves, which its epithet *aquefolium* means. The plant is native to the Pacific Northwest, and the berries were eaten by aboriginal inhabitants and are sometimes made into jams. Native herbalists used the berries to treat stomach upset, and extracts have been effective against skin disorders, particularly eczema and psoriasis. The root and bark of the stem are also recommended as an alternative to goldenseal for infections of the mucous membranes, taken as tinctures or capsules but not during pregnancy.

Passionflower *(Passiflora incarnata)* refers to a genus of flowering plants, some of which are vines and others shrubs. There are many species native to North and South America, Australia and New Zealand and Eastern and Southern Asia, and 2 new species have been described in the last decade. They tend to flower in the spring, and derive their name from the Easter season. The plants are food for many types of butterfly, produce nectar that feeds several kinds of hummingbirds and have evolved in tandem with large bees that are uniquely able to pollinate the flowers. Passionflower species are widely cultivated for their beautiful flowers, and the fruit is edible and often used for juice. The leaves and roots of a North American variety were used by native herbalists for a calming tea, utilized for insomnia, epilepsy and psychiatric agitation. An extract of the plant compared favorably to oxazepam in the treatment of generalized anxiety, and passionflower is listed in the European Pharmacopeia, which recommends preparations standardized to contain at least 1.5 per cent vitexin, a potent antioxidant. Modern herbal medicine utilizes the flowers for tinctures, teas and capsules, and recommends passionflower for anxiety, heart palpitations, insomnia and restlessness with few if any adverse effects.

Pau d'arco (*Tabebuia aellanedae* or *impestiginosa*) is a Portuguese name for trees and shrubs sometimes called roble or trumpet tree. It is native to Mexico, Cuba, Hispaniola, Brazil and Argentina, and is an important source of wood that is light and resistant to salt, air and water. The bark of one species is used to make the psychedelic drink Ayahuasca, sometimes used in South American cultures to induce mystical or religious experiences. It has been used by native and medical herbalists as a cancer treatment; other medicinal uses for teas made from the bark or capsules containing ground bark are parasitic and fungal infections, particularly *Candida*, and prostatitis. It should be avoided during pregnancy and breastfeeding because of its potential psychedelic and cytotoxic effects, and because large doses can cause nausea, digestive upset and bleeding.

***Peppermint** (Mentha piperita)* is a hybrid of watermint and spearmint, and was described and named in Latin by Linnaeus himself in 1753. It was first developed in Europe, but as a hybrid can grow almost anywhere, and is universally used as a source of mint flavoring. The plant is very high in menthol content, which is responsible for the cool sensation on application of peppermint oil. The flowers produce a great deal of nectar, and if foraged by bees can produce a very flavorful honey. Peppermint has been used medicinally for up to 10,000 years, generally for abdominal and digestive problems, although there is evidence that peppermint protects against the effects of radiation therapy for cancer and may enhance memory and alertness, for which it is used in aromatherapy. Peppermint oil is approved in Italy for the treatment of irritable bowel syndrome, and the German Commission E has supported its medical use as an anodyne, antibacterial, anticatarrhal, anti-inflammatory, antispasmodic, carminative, cholagogue, cooling and secretolytic agent. Tinctures, teas and essential oil from the leaves are generally recommended for colic, fever, gallstones, headache, indigestion, irritable bowel symptoms and nausea, and the main side effect is heartburn from the oil. Infants and young children may develop apnea and respiratory distress if peppermint oil is applied topically to the face or nose.

Plantain (Musa x paradisica) are the members along with bananas of the genus *Musa*. Whereas bananas can be eaten raw, plantains generally require cooking and are usually the hybrid of 2 wild species, *Musa accuminata* and *Musa balbisiana*. Plantains originated in Southeast Asia and Oceania, but are now a food staple in Africa, the Caribbean, Central America and parts of South America as well, and are also used to make beer. Plantains are rich in potassium and fiber, and have more starch and less sugar than bananas, which is why they must be processed before eating. The very large and sturdy leaves can serve as plates or to wrap food for cooking, and the shoot can be chopped and used in salads and curries that are thought to improve digestion and prevent kidney stones. Juice from the stem and peel is also used for first aid for burns, abrasions and insect bites. Tinctures applied topically or taken by mouth along with tea made from chopped leaves are prescribed as an antiseptic and anti-inflammatory, and for infections of the respiratory and urinary tracts. Adverse effects have not been encountered.

Pygeum *(Pygeum africanum)* is an extract from the bark of the red stinkwood *(Prunus africanus)*, an evergreen tree that grows in mountainous parts of sub-Saharan Africa and its adjacent islands. The bark of the tree has long been used in traditional medicine there. The National Standard Research Collaboration, which reviews the clinical evidence for and against the effectiveness of natural or alternative therapies, has concluded that pygeum moderately improves the urinary symptoms caused by prostate enlargement, although it does not shrink the prostate gland or reverse the process of benign prostatic hypertrophy in older men. Pygeum apparently contains inhibitors of prostaglandin, which initiates urinary tract inflammation that precipitates the symptoms of urinary hesitancy, frequency and urgency, and can be taken as a tincture or in tablets or capsules. There are no adverse effects except occasional digestive upset. Pygeum is often taken in combination with saw palmetto to enhance prostate health.

Red Raspberry *(Rubus idaeus)* is the edible fruit of several members of the rose family, which has one of the highest fiber contents of any food, as much as 6 per cent of total weight. Raspberries also contain large amounts of vitamin C and manganese, moderate amounts of vitamin K and have a low sugar content and glycemic index. Many different antioxidants and compounds effective against cell proliferation, and therefore potentially useful against cancer, are present in the fruits. In addition to their food value, tinctures and teas from raspberries and their leaves are astringent and calming, and have long been used as a uterine tonic before and during pregnancy, and for the regulation of abnormal menses. Diarrhea, nausea and vomiting and sore throat have also been treated, usually without ill effects.

Reishi *(Ganoderma lucidum)* is the Japanese name for the "supernatural mushroom", called *lingzhi* in China, *yeong ji* in Korea and *linh chi* in Vietnam. It is the oldest medicinal mushroom, having been introduced in traditional Chinese practice about 2000 years ago. The mushroom has been thought to sharpen the wits, lighten the body and prolong life, and different types or colors of *lingzhi* were thought to differentially benefit the liver (green), heart (red), spleen (yellow), lung (white), kidney (black) and general life essence (purple). Ganodermic acids are the main active ingredients, and these principally affect the immune system and possibly influence the regeneration of liver cells and amount or distribution of some neurotransmitters. Eating the mushroom, drinking decoctions of its roots or using tinctures of the fruiting body or capsules with powdered mushroom has been recommended for allergies, bronchitis, adjunctive cancer treatment, support of the immune system during and after chemotherapy or radiation treatment, general detoxification, hepatitis and support of liver function, hypertension and memory disorders. There are generally no adverse effects, but caution is needed during pregnancy because some of the many alkaloids in the mushroom can have toxic effects.

Rosemary *(Rosemarinus officinalis)* is a perennial Mediterranean herb with needle-like leaves that is a member of the mint family. It was said to have been draped around the shoulders of the goddess Aphrodite after she rose from the sea, and came to be called "rose of Mary" because the Virgin Mary placed her blue cloak over a white bush when she rested, and the flowers turned blue and have remained so. It is a popular ornamental plant, is used in fragrances and is widely used in Mediterranean cooking; it is a good source of vitamin B_6, iron and calcium, and prevents oils containing *omega*-3 fatty acids from becoming rancid. It has been used as a wedding decoration and love charm since ancient times, and was thought in the Middle Ages to be useful in divination. It was sometimes thrown into graves as a gesture of remembrance for the dead, and came to be associated with memory function for that reason. Ophelia in *Hamlet* says that rosemary is for remembrance, and Don Quixote uses it in the Cervantes novel to mix the miraculous balm of Fierabras. Queen Elizabeth of Hungary is credited with mixing fresh rosemary, wine and spirits to create Hungary Water, used to treat paralysis and gout, and antioxidants and camphor have been isolated the plant, along with an essential oil important in aromatherapy. The leaves can be steeped to make tea or tinctures, or rosemary can be added to various herbal formulas according to the conditions treated. The current herbal medicine recommendations are usually for antioxidant protection, *Candida* infection, hypothyroidism, infestation with lice, memory disorders and as a general nervous system tonic and calmative. It should be avoided during pregnancy, but is otherwise felt safe.

Sage (*Salvia officinalis*) is another mint relative native to the Mediterranean and long used for cooking and healing. Like many other plants called *officinalis*, sage was named for its medical use: medicinal herbs were kept and compounded in the storeroom maintained for that purpose in a monastery, the *officina.* The ancient Greeks used it for snakebite and infertility, while the Romans found it to be a useful diuretic, as well as a local anesthetic for the skin and a styptic, which stops bleeding by constricting blood vessels in the skin. It was one of four herbs used in Marseilles or Four Thieves Vinegar, supposedly divulged by 4 graverobbers arrested during an outbreak of plague, who were spared from execution in return for the secret of this concoction intended to prevent the Black Death. In both Indian and European herbal traditions, sage has been used for respiratory and gastrointestinal disorders, as well as an antibiotic, antifungal, antispasmodic anti-sweating agent, estrogen analogue, hypoglycemic and general tonic. The herb has a strong drying quality. Sage extract has been shown to improve mild-to-moderate Alzheimer's disease and to lower elevated levels of cholesterol and triglycerides. Its essential oil contains the psychoactive terpene thujone, which is also present in absinthe, and vitamin B_3 (niacin and nicotinamide), chlorogenic and caffeic acids which slow the entry of glucose into the blood after a meal, the *omega*-9 fatty acid oleic acid and antioxidant tannins and flavonoids are in leaf extracts. Teas and tinctures from the leaves are used to dry up excessive secretions and stop inappropriate breast milk production (galactorrhea), alleviate gas and hot flashes and relieve sore throat and gum inflammation. Use for more than 2 weeks has rarely caused neurological symptoms.

Sarsparilla *(Smilax regelii, aristolochifolia* or *aspera)* was once in the United States Pharmacopoeia as a treatment for syphilis, and has been recommended for arthritis and leprosy among other conditions. This group of Central American and Caribbean plants was used by native herbalists, and was recommended in the 19th century to induce sweating, but came to be used chiefly for the soft drink sarsaparilla, an antecedent of modern root beer. Extracts of the root have antioxidant properties, but current practice focuses on acne, eczema and psoriasis, treated with topical tinctures or oral capsule, watching for stomach upset and avoiding its use during pregnancy.

Saw palmetto *(Serenoa repens* or *Sabal serrulata)* is one of the most widely used herbal remedies, being shown effective for prostate enlargement in many studies. The first Latin name refers to a small palm tree that grows in the Southeastern and South Central United States and may live 500 to 700 years; *S. serrulata* is a larger palm tree that grows in the Caribbean and in Central and South America. Edible hearts of palm come from *S. serrulata,* while the North American tree is more bitter and is more often eaten by butterfly larvae than people. The fruits of both are rich in fatty acids and plant sterols, and saw palmetto extracts have been in several large studies as effective or more effective as pharmaceutical drugs in alleviating urinary symptoms and forestalling the need for surgery for benign prostatic hypertrophy. The berries are used to make tinctures, teas or capsules that are also used for acne, baldness in men and polycystic ovarian disease in women, attended occasionally by stomach upset but to be avoided during pregnancy and breastfeeding.

Senna *(Cassia senna)* is a member of the *Fabaceae* family, which includes beans and peas. The plants are mostly used in landscaping, but cassia gum, from the seeds of Chinese cassia, is a thickening agent, neutral henna from Italian cassia is used as a hair treatment and the leaves and flowers of Siamese cassia are used in Thai cooking. Alexandrian senna has been used as a laxative since the days of ancient Egypt, and glycosides specific to these plants, called sennosides, have been shown to induce fluid secretion in the large intestine and vigorous contractions of the walls of the colon, making them a strong stimulant laxative. Some senna plants also produce resveratrol to protect them against bacterial or fungal attack; this compound is prominent in grape juice and wine also, and is thought to cause or assist weight loss. The senna leaves and pods are ground to produce capsules, suppositories and tablets for laxative use, or can be taken as tea or tincture, but with chronic use can cause bowel sluggishness or diarrhea. They should not be taken over long periods, and must be avoided in cases of bowel obstruction.

Shiitake *(Lentinus edodes)* is an Asian edible mushroom that has been cultivated in China since the 1st century A.D., and is also widely used in Japan, Korea and Thailand, particularly for miso soup and vegetarian dishes. Shiitake has been used medicinally to enhance *qi* and to retard the aging process, and has been prescribed particularly for exhaustion and weakness, poor circulation, liver disease and upper respiratory problems. Active Hexose Correlated Compound (AHCC) isolated from the mushroom is the second most commonly used alternative medicine in Japan, and is prescribed for cancer treatment because it increases the numbers and effect of killer lymphocytes. Eritadenene inhibits the production of homocysteine and may therefore lessen the oxidation of cholesterol and initiation of atherosclerosis. These compounds, particularly AHCC, also enhance the activity of the immune system and may assist in fighting infection. In western herbalism, food use or drops of tincture of the fruiting body are recommended for bronchitis, adjunctive cancer treatment, hepatitis, HIV infection and general immune support, with rare digestive upset being reported.

Skullcap *(Scutellaria lateriflora* or *galericulata)* is a perennial herb widely distributed in the Northern Hemisphere and part of the mint family. Skullcap is widely used in herbalism for anxiety, agitation and indigestion, but native North American healers used the blue skullcap (*S. lateriflora*) and European herbalists used the common skullcap (*S. galereticulata*). Western and Southern skullcap are sometimes used medicinally as well, and are genetically, chemically and therapeutically similar. Drinking the teas and tinctures, smoking the dried leaf, and taking capsules or tablets have all been recommended for the plant's sedative, anxiety-relieving and diuretic properties. The main chemical constituents are baicalin, a flavonoid that has antioxidant effects and also works on the GABA receptors involved in anxiety, which is present in the leaf, and in the rest of the plant, chrysin and tannin, which are antioxidant flavonoids that may have some estrogen-like effects. Modern herbalists recommend extracts of the above-ground aerial parts of the plant, prepared as tinctures, teas or capsules, for anxiety, digestive problems, hyperactivity and insomnia, generally without adverse effects.

Slippery Elm (*Ulmus fulva* or *rubra*) is a North American elm tree sometimes called red elm. Its wood was used to make the yoke of the Liberty Bell, and was also important in the construction of covered wagons and wagon wheels for the settling of the West. The slippery elm has been less severely affected by Dutch elm disease than other American elms, but has been damaged by the elm leaf beetle. The inner bark of the tree contains mucilage, and has been used as a demulcent since colonial times, while powdered leaves and bark have been used for teas for digestive upset and skin disorders, particularly psoriasis. Current herbal practice recognizes tinctures, tablets, capsules and lozenges made from the inner bark as effective for conditions that irritate the mucous membranes of the digestive, respiratory and urinary tracts, with few if any side effects.

Soy (*Glycine max*) is a legume almost universally cultivated for food and has many medicinal uses, particularly with respect to estrogen and its effects, but is attended by some risks of allergy as well. Soybean oil and protein account for about 60 per cent of the weight of dry soybeans, and the protein is mostly heat-stable and easily stored. The 35 per cent carbohydrate content is mostly fiber and its sugars are mostly simple ones. Soybean oil contains predominantly unsaturated fats and the proportion of essential fatty acids is relatively high. There are also plant steroid and estrogen analogues, and antioxidant flavonoids. These are all beneficial for cardiovascular health and hormonal balance, especially women, and some soy proteins may have anticancer effects. Soy allergy is relatively common, however, and repeated soy exposure may trigger intolerance and food sensitivity, especially in children. There has been concern that soy products, particularly isoflavones, may be linked to certain types of cancer, and that soy products may worsen gout or hypothyroidism, so soy should be avoided by those with cancer, gout and thyroid disease. Otherwise, capsules, tablets and powder derived from the beans have been recommended for cancer prevention as opposed to treatment; elevated cholesterol and triglycerides, menopausal symptoms, osteoporosis and premenstrual syndrome, with digestive upset the main adverse effect.

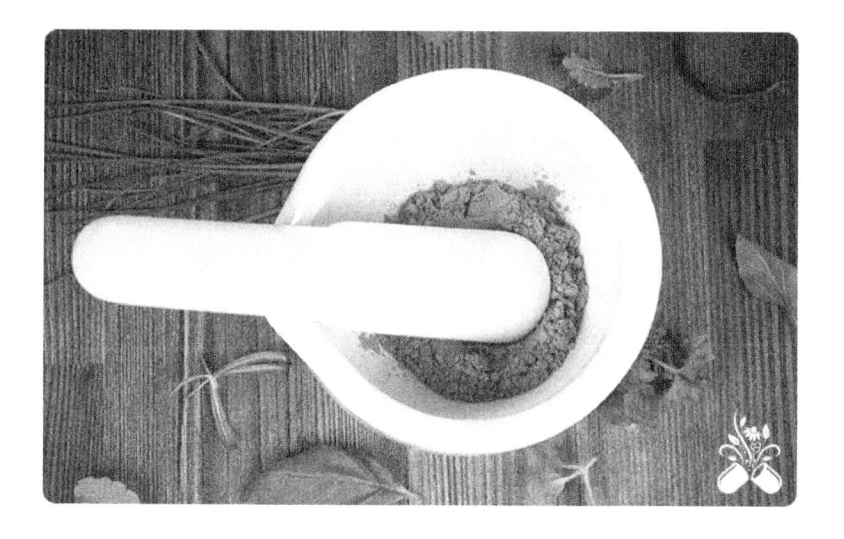

Spirulina *(Anthospira maxima* or *platensis)* are actually bacteria rather than plants, but have the capacity for photosynthesis to make food as plants do. *Cyanobacteria* such as the *Anthospira* are thought to have been an important factor in the emergence of animal life by producing oxygen through their metabolism and changing the reducing atmosphere of the primordial Earth to an oxidizing one, thereby making biodiversity possible. They were a food source in ancient times for American and African natives, and cakes of *tecuitlatl* were described by Cortez and his soldiers on their arrival in Mexico. Spirulina consists mostly of protein (up to 70 per cent), and has all amino acids, all essential fatty acids, all minerals that may need to be supplemented, and almost all necessary vitamins (the B_{12} in spirulina is biologically inactive in humans). There are multiple beneficial pigments and proteins as well. It is thus considered a "superfood" and has no apparent toxicity, but in some cases may have biological contaminants such as lead, mercury and arsenic or toxic algae, so a pure and uncontaminated preparation of domestic origin is safest. Spirulina also contains high levels of vitamin K and phenylalanine, and therefore can cause problems for those taking anticoagulants or people with the genetic disorder phenylketonuria. Its main use in herbal medicine is as a nutritional supplement and aid to detoxification, and it can be taken as tablets and capsules or mixed as powder in food and drinks. Anemia, adjunctive cancer treatment, high cholesterol, immune support and alleviation of the toxic effects of radiation are recommended uses.

Saint John's Wort *(Hypericum perforatum)* has long been used for pain, injuries and burns; King George V of England was so impressed with its efficacy for hunting and riding injuries that he named one of his race horses Hypericum. Hypericum is actually a genus of some 500 flowering plants, many of which are weeds and grow almost everywhere in the world but deserts and polar regions. King Mithridates of Pontus (now in Turkey) experimented with poisons and antidotes on his prisoners during the 1st century BCE, and developed "mithridatium", which contained opium, castor and myrrh as well as hypericum. The Greco-Roman herbalist Celsus advocated hypericum as the basis of a theriac or general panacea about a century later, and both Chinese and European physicians developed multi-ingredient healing potions, usually including hypericum but also opiates, in ensuing centuries, and such medicines came to be known as Venice treacle in England. The oil of hypericum has been used in folk medicine in many countries, and hyperforin and hypericin haven been isolated from the plant and shown to have wound-healing but also moderate antidepressant properties, probably through the enhancement of serotonin levels or effect. Tinctures or capsules are made from the flowers and the oil can be applied topically for abrasions, bruises, burns, and the pain of nerve injury or irritation. Anxiety, mild to moderate depression and seasonal affective disorder have been successfully treated, but sensitization to sunlight should be watched for and St. John's Wort should not be taken together with pharmaceutical antidepressants.

Tea tree *(Melaleuca alternifolia)* refers to several Australian and New Zealand shrubs in the myrtle family. The name comes from Captain James Cook, whose men used the leaves to make a tea substitute during South Sea explorations. Australian chemist Arthur Penfold studied the essential oil from the leaves in the 1920s, found it to be a powerful antiseptic and later demonstrated its use in aromatherapy. Approximately 100 chemical compounds have been isolated from the leaves, chiefly terpenes that are very much like camphor, and that are toxic if taken internally and often irritating to the skin. The tincture of the leaves can be used as a mouthwash but should not be swallowed. Topical application of the oil is recommended for acne, burns, fungal infections like athlete's foot, other skin infections, vaginitis and warts.

Thuja *(Thuja occidentalis)* was once called *arborvitae*, the tree of life, but has been thought to have dangerous and even lethal components, particularly the terpene thujone, which was at one time an ingredient in absinthe and has been alleged to be the reason the painter Vincent Van Gogh cut off his ear and later committed suicide. Thujone was probably not the reason and absinthe, which was for a time banned, has again been legalized with the thujone removed. Thujone is a potent antagonist of the GABA receptor, and other potentially toxic alkaloids have made thuja potentially useful as a wart treatment. This is the main medical use of the essential oil or tincture of the bark and leaves, and it should not be taken internally.

Thyme *(Thyme vulgaris)* is a spice in the mint family that is an essential part of many cuisines, and was used by the Egyptians for embalming, the Greeks for baths and incense and the Romans for purification and flavoring. Thyme incensed over the deceased or placed in coffins has been thought to ease the passage into the next world, and the essential oil (thymol) is widely used in sanitizers, disinfectants and mouthwashes. The leaves and flowers can also be used for tinctures, teas or capsules, and these are recommended for respiratory and urinary tract infections, while the oil can be applied topically for skin fungus. Abdominal pain can be a side effect of too much essential oil.

Turmeric *(Curcuma longa)* is a member of the ginger family that is an important ingredient in East Asian and Middle Eastern food. It was early imported into Europe and was called "Indian saffron" because it resembled saffron but was (and is) much less expensive. The Siddha system of medicine in South India and Sri Lanka has used turmeric since the 2nd millennium BCE for stomach and liver ailments, skin conditions and as an antimicrobial agent, while traditional Chinese medicine views it as an antiseptic and agent for various types of infection. Much recent research suggests that the principal ingredient, curcumin, is an antioxidant, antibacterial and antiviral agent and has anticancer effects. The rhizome, the above ground part of the plant, can be ground for capsules or made into a tincture, and this is recommended for arthritis, digestive disorders, inflammation and possibly as an adjunct to cancer treatment. Turmeric is a cholagogue, so should be used with caution if gallstones are present, and its possible cell toxicity as an anticancer agent suggests that only low doses should be used during pregnancy.

Usnea *(Usnea barbata)* is a lichen also known as tree moss or old man's beard. Lichens represent the symbiosis of a fungus and an alga, the fungus in this case being one of the *Ascomycota* while the alga is a chlorophyte, one of the exceedingly numerous green algae. Usnea grows on trees, and has been used medicinally for about 2000 years. It is used in cosmetics and dyes, and is effective against various fish infections in ponds and aquariums. Usnic acid derived from the lichen is an effective antibiotic and antifungal compound, and the hairlike structure of the lichen allowed it to be applied to surface wounds as a dressing. Usnea is also high in vitamin C. It is currently used as an antibiotic for lung, respiratory tract and urinary tract infections, and is approved by the German Commission E for oral and throat infections. There have been concerns about liver toxicity, so tinctures or capsules prepared from the whole lichen should be used with caution in those with liver problems and by pregnant or breastfeeding women.

Uva ursi *(Arctostaphylos uva ursi)* is known as "bearberry" or "bear grapes", because its fruit is very attractive to bears. It is widely distributed in northern climates, and has long been used as a diuretic and antimicrobial agent, and Native Americans smoked its dried leaves for health and possibly narcotic or stimulant effects. The glycoside arbutin, obtained from the leaves, is a diuretic and antimicrobial, but some of its hydroquinone constituents may be toxic to the liver in undiluted form. The leaves are currently used for tinctures or capsules that are recommended for urinary tract infections and prevention of kidney stones, but excessive or chronic use may cause abdominal cramping, nausea or vomiting.

Valerian *(Valeriana officinalis)* is a sweet-smelling flowering herb found in Europe and Asia, and used as a calmative and sedative by Hippocrates and Galen as well as their followers. It contains the inhibitory transmitter GABA itself, as well as alkaloids and valerenic acid which have actions on the $GABA_A$ receptors of the brain that are similar to those of the benzodiazepine drugs. It is sold as a nutritional supplement in the United States, due to insufficient evidence of efficacy to satisfy the FDA, but in other countries it is widely prescribed for sleep disorders, anxiety, pain and cramping as well as other digestive symptoms of anxious origin and as a muscle relaxant. The root is usually ground for tinctures or to put in capsules for these uses, and the main adverse effect is occasional morning drowsiness.

Vitex *(Vitex agnus-castus)* or chasteberry got its common name from its early use as an anaphrodisiac, to lessen sexual desire. Pliny the Elder reported its use during the Athenian *Thesmophoria*, when women customarily left their husbands' beds and remained chaste for a time. Its calming effects are described in the writings of Chaucer, and it was sometimes called "monk's pepper" in the belief that monks could use it for medicinal preparations to foster chastity. Later chemical studies found flavonoids and alkaloids that may work on the endocrine system, particularly the pituitary gland, as well as steroid-like hormones that can influence the dopamine system and thus possibly behavior in addition to reducing prolactin levels, which can lessen estrogen and progesterone production in women and release of testosterone in men. There is evidence of effectiveness and safety from controlled trials in premenstrual syndrome, cyclical breast pain, hyperprolactinemia (elevated prolactin levels with inappropriate lactation in women and infertility in men and women) and luteal phase defect (infertility due to this stage of the menstrual cycle being too short to allow embryos to implant). Some clinical evidence suggests effect and safety in polycystic ovarian syndrome and bleeding due to uterine fibroids. There are suggestions that vitex may also alleviate menstrual symptoms and help those of prostatism. The dried fruit is used for tinctures, teas, capsules or tablets, but should not be combined with birth control pills and ought to be taken under the supervision of a physician versed in herbal medicine during pregnancy. Digestive upset, headaches and skin rash are occasional side effects.

Willow *(Salix alba)* is one of some 400 species of tree mostly found in the Northern Hemisphere. It is of great historical importance in herbal medicine, because the precursors of aspirin were derived from its bark and this led to the development of the drug in the 19th century. Willow bark and leaves were used for fever and pain in ancient Egypt, and this was another remedy prescribed by Hippocrates. It was a staple of native American healing, and clinical studies of its effects were presented to the Royal Society in London in 1763. Salicin, the active ingredient, was purified in 1828, and it was recognized as a precursor of salicylic acid with anti-inflammatory effect. Willow is also important for agriculture as a source of nectar and pollen for bees, in art as the source of charcoal for drawing and willow rods for sculpture and weaving, as a source of biomass fuel in Europe and the United States and is one of the "four species" used ritually during the Jewish holiday of Sukkot as well as the attribute of the Buddhist *bodhisattva* of compassion, Kwan Yin. The bark is usually prepared as tincture or tea, or put into capsules, and is recommended as a natural alternative to anti-inflammatory drugs for arthritis, fever, headache or other types of pain. It can impair immune defense during viral infections, and may cause bleeding in people taking anticoagulants, so should be avoided in these circumstances.

Witch Hazel *(Hammamelis virginiana)* refers to 3 species of flowering shrubs that grow in Japan, China and North America; the American form is sometimes called winterbloom. It contains many phenols and a modest amount of essential oil that are strongly astringent, and ancient North American native healers prepared a decoction for inflammation, swelling and tumors, which was adopted by the Pilgrims and later colonists. Dr. Charles Hawes of Connecticut developed a means of distilling the bark with steam, and Hawes Extract began to be produced in 1846 and has been manufactured by the same family in Connecticut since that time. Witch hazel should not be used internally or it will cause severe stomach cramping, but as a topical tincture it can be applied to eczema, cold sores and inflamed gums, and is particularly recommended to facilitate wound healing and shrink hemorrhoids and varicose veins.

Yerba santa *(Eryodiction californicum)* means "sacred herb", and the California and Oregon plant is sometimes also called mountain balm. The leaves have an unpleasant odor and a bitter taste, so the plant has generally been safe from animals, although insects like the leaves and butterflies seek the nectar. It is also adapted to fire and is one of the first species to sprout after a wildfire, and so is used for revegetation of damaged or disturbed areas. The leaves produce 4 flavones that diminish bitter tastes and are used in the food and pharmaceutical industry. Preparations of the dried leaves facilitate the expulsion of mucus, and are used for respiratory infections, and the leaves can be applied to the skin in a poultice to relieve joint pain or lessen inflammation around bites, stings and wounds. There are no reported adverse effects.

Chapter 5

FLOWER REMEDIES

Another form of herbal medicine involves preparations of flower essence made by suspending various flowers in water for several hours then collecting and bottling the water or making an alcohol-based tincture of the flower with water. The best known of these preparations are 38 essences developed in the 1930s by Dr. Edward Bach (he pronounced it "batch"), a British physician and bacteriologist who miraculously recovered after the resection of a malignant abdominal tumor and devoted the remainder of his life to homeopathic medicine and a search for a natural method of treating the whole person. Bach concluded that a patient's spiritual and emotional state determined whether and how completely recovery from illness would occur, and found that the essences of wildflowers collected on the Oxfordshire farm to which he retired after closing his lucrative London practice could affect the necessary emotional change. Dr. Richard Katz in California further refined the Bach system in the 1970s (Flower Essence System), and Australian herbalist Ian White has derived a collection of 69 therapeutic essences from bush flowers on that continent.

The view of most natural medicine practitioners who use flower essence therapies is that people are better able to manage various medical problems, have fewer stress-related problems and complications and feel and function better despite their illness if they are as free as possible from emotional upset and conflict. In addition, many conditions manifest themselves at times of stress, and may be forestalled by alleviation of such mental influences. Flower essences work by allowing suppressed emotions and conflicts to be expressed and resolved, and are thought to help addiction by alleviating chronic emotional upset that triggers cravings and use. Bach combined 5 essences in a combination product that remains the best-selling alternative medicine product on the market in the United Kingdom: *Rescue Remedy* contains *cherry plum* to foster calmness and determination, *clematis* for clear thinking, *impatiens* to instill patience, *rock rose* that antagonizes fear and panic, and *star of Bethlehem* to alleviate emotional trauma. It can be used as psychological "first aid" in any stressful situation, by placing 2 drops on the tongue or in a glass of water; a drop can also be applied at the wrist or on the forehead at a time of crisis. Flower remedies can be customized by combining up to 6 commercially-available essences in a one-ounce dropper bottle of amber glass, diluting with spring water and then putting 4 drops of the mixture on the tongue up to four times a day; a bedtime dose helps with the restless sleep and dream disturbance that may come with quitting any addiction. Flower remedies may also be made at home with freshly picked flowers, spring water and apple cider vinegar.

The flower essences work by alleviating emotional states that are not conducive to health, and work on particular personality types and psychological constitutions for each flower. Many of the characteristics listed below are negative, but these profiles are not intended to be pejorative; the idea is that people who are for whatever reason fearful or unhappy or preoccupied may have more trouble with various illness, and that improving fear or unhappiness or preoccupation will make it easier to treat them.

People who will improve with *Agrimony* are apprehensive, cover up distress and attempt to hide problems from themselves and others. *Aspen* will help people who are anxious and apprehensive, and are vaguely fearful about things they cannot name.

Beech works for people who are analytical and critical of themselves and others, tending at times to be judgmental and less tolerant of others than they might be.
Those who respond to *Centaury* cannot say "no" to others and are sometimes exploited by other people because they are overly anxious to please.

Cerato candidates are often indecisive and need confirmation from others before making their own judgments, about which they are uncertain.

Cherry Plum helps people who are afraid of losing control and doing terrible things, or who are sometimes irrational or have fears of losing their minds.

The **Chestnut Bud** person seemingly cannot learn from experience, and makes the same mistakes again and again.

Chicory is for those who are self-centered and possessive, who may be overly protective of others or try to manipulate them.

Clematis, which is in Rescue Remedy, energizes and focuses people who are absent-minded, disinterested or inclined to daydream or sleep.

Crab Apple is the "cleaning remedy" and helps with detoxification from illness or with concerns about being unclean or unhygienic.

People who need ***Elm*** take on too much and are then overwhelmed, and are prone to general feelings of depression.

Those who need ***Gentian*** are negative and depressed, but know exactly what they are depressed about. They are often despondent about overcoming their problems, and are pessimistic about surmounting specific obstacles or difficulties.

Gorse candidates are despondent and pessimistic about things in general, and have given up hope.

Heather helps people who are lonely, needy and preoccupied with their own problems; they will often talk at great length about their unhappiness.

People helped by ***Holly*** are sharp-tongued like the points of a holly leaf, and often feel spiteful, resentful or envious.

Those who feel better with **Honeysuckle** tend to be wistful and nostalgic, and dwell in conversation on past happiness or unhappiness.

Hornbeam is helpful for people who are physically or mentally tired, and for procrastinators.

Impatiens works on impatience by itself and in the rescue combination, as the name implies: people who are themselves quick in thought and action but are irritated by those who are not will often feel better after using this essence.

Larch helps those with an inferiority complex, who expect failure in their daily situations and in confronting illnesses.

"Worriers", shy and timid people and those who have specific fears about everyday life will feel better with **Mimulus**.

People who are miserable and sorrowful for no reason and periodically experience depression or hopelessness, who feel that there is a dark cloud overhead, are likely to respond to **Mustard Seed.**

Oak helps stoic people and workaholics, who seem as stout and strong as the tree but insist on confronting obstacles and health problems entirely on their own, sometimes at great cost.

The **Olive** person is the reverse, drained and exhausted by problems or illnesses, out of steam and at wit's end.

Pine assists perfectionists, people dissatisfied with themselves and those prone to guilt and apology in dealing with problems and illnesses.

Those who anticipate misfortune for themselves, fear that the worst will happen to others and project worry may do better with ***Red Chestnut.***

Rock Rose, a constituent of Rescue Remedy, is itself a useful essence for emergencies in people prone to panic attacks or who respond catastrophically to illnesses and accidents.

Rock Water candidates are opinionated, more critical of others than of themselves, puritanical and austere.

Scleranthus helps people who are vacillating and indecisive or have changeable moods and often feel out of sorts; this has also been used for premenstrual syndrome and various illnesses and symptoms aggravated by menses.

Star of Bethlehem, the final component of the rescue preparation, is a "comfort remedy", for people who are devastated and inconsolable on account of illness or problems.

Sweet Chestnut helps those who are dejected, anguished and feel pushed to their limits.

Enthusiastic or highly-strung people, who may not be able to see beyond their current concern or situation, or who are workaholics or determined to overcome an illness, will do better with *Vervain*.

Vine helps people who are capable and confident but may be rigid or "bossy", often effective leaders but determined to have their own way even when ill.

Walnut helps people feel better, and may avoid exacerbation of illnesses, when they are undergoing change or transition, such as divorce, relocation or menopause.

Water Violet candidates may be calming to others but not always calm themselves; they are often gentle and quiet "loners".

Those helped by **White Chestnut,** on the other hand, are often in turmoil, worriers and insomniacs who feel that their minds are racing.

Wild Oats is helpful for people who feel that life is passing them by, but who may be indecisive or ambivalent about how to change this.

Willow will help people who feel that life is unjust or they have been wronged, tend to blame others for their misfortunes and may be resentful and unforgiving.

Conclusion

The history of medical use of plants and their component parts and chemical contents is very long. Herbs figure importantly in the ancient medical literature of the East, Middle East and North America, and were the mainstays of classical Greek and Roman medicine. Most of the classical medical literature that survived into the Middle Ages was related to herbal treatments, and another large component of plant-related medicine was preserved by the physicians of the Islamic world during the Dark Ages.

The development in recent centuries of pharmaceutical drugs, which were sometimes cheaper to manufacture, easier to standardize as to ingredients and preparation and less attended by toxic effect, was both a confirmation of the importance of plant remedies in human medicine and a turn away from patient-centered and ecologically-sensitive medical treatment. With time, the potential problems occasioned by complete reliance on scientific medical practice and surgical and pharmaceutical drug treatment have been recognized, and the various doctrines and schools of holistic medicine have helped to restore some balance. At the same time, the growing interest in medicinal use of plants and herbs has in some cases led to the overuse and overharvesting of some medicinal plants which are now endangered, and the problems of habitat reduction and change can affect therapeutic herbs as well as other plants and animals.

There is also growing recognition of the potential for sensitivity and allergy to many plant products, and of the many possibilities for interaction between plant products and pharmaceutical drugs as well as interactions between different plant products. This makes it important for those who would grow and use medicinal plants for themselves to learn the basics of plant toxicology and pharmacology, and to correctly identify one plant from another and tell beneficial ones from harmful ones. It is also advisable for people with medical conditions and illnesses to consult at least initially with medical herbalists, natural medicine practitioners or physicians with expertise in complementary or alternative medicine in order to use most safely some of the plant-based alternatives.

FURTHER READING

Balch JF, Stengler M. *Prescriptions for Natural Cures, ed. 2.* Hoboken, NJ, John Wiley and Sons, 2010.

Balch PA, Bell S. *Prescription for Dietary t, ed. 2.* New York, Penguin-Avery, 2012.

Chevallier A. *Encyclopedia of Herbal Medicine: The Definitive Home Reference Guide to 550 Key Herbs with all their Uses as Remedies for Common Ailments.* New York, DK, 2000.

Hoffman D. *Medical Herbalism: The Science, Principles and Practices of Herbal Medicine.* Rochester, VT, Healing Arts Press, 2003.

Stengler M. *The Natural Physician's Hee aling Therapies.* New York, Prentice Hall, 2010.

Printed in Great Britain
by Amazon